To
Petu

In memory of
Dwight Russell Ten Broeck

Acknowledgements

Thanks to a great team. The book would be a poorer version without the help and guidance of any one of you.

I could not have been more fortunate in my editorial team: Hilary Herbold, Stephanie Daval, Romi Mukerjee, and Melisa Baez.

In their own ways and in varying degrees they have enriched as well as expertly edited the manuscript. Each has been of fundamental value.

Thanks to my older daughter Paula, whose insights and confidences she felt comfortable enough to share with her dad, and who by her conduct in this life gives me the validation to continue saying what I have to say.

Thanks to my younger daughter Caty for similarly wonderful reasons and for the artwork that generationally connects the reader to the words.

It is ironic how often our own shit detectors get clogged with our own shit. Thanks to my wife Jacalyn. Every would-be genius needs a Petu to regularly set them straight. In this regard I have been most fortunate.

Table of Contents

Introduction

This is a book for coming-of-agers, 18-25 years-old, who are open to life's possibilities. It is, in some ways, too broad of an audience. I have directed it to this age group because, by 18, it is certainly time to begin to find your own reality, and at 25 there is still time to figure it out. Because of the broad audience, some things that are said may seem difficult to one reader, while other parts may seem simple to another.

I have tried to write about the things in life that you can't get a straight answer to. I don't know if I've done it better than anyone else because I don't know if anyone else has really tried.

I have tried, and I hope that it is helpful to you.

> *"The vanity of teaching often tempteth a man to forget he is a blockhead."*
>
> George Savile, 1st Marquis of Halifax, 1633-95

The More Things Change…

"It is a civilization which has destroyed the simplicity and repose of life; replaced its contentment, its poetry, its soft romance-dreams and visions with the money-fever, sordid ideals, vulgar ambitions, and the sleep which does not refresh; it has invented a thousand useless luxuries, and turned them into necessities, it has created a thousand vicious appetites and satisfies none of them; it has dethroned God and set up a shekel in His place."

Mark Twain, circa 1885

On Becoming Yourself

Most of us aren't very sure when we're young, can't be very sure, how we want to be in ten, twenty, or thirty years. Many of the influential people in our lives we have yet to meet. Some of the most important aren't even on the drawing board. Life is unpredictable. Toss in the bursting menu of opportunity available to coming-of-agers these days, and it becomes pretty clear that "becoming yourself" is a process best taken one day at a time.

There are lots of things that you can do in the meantime: Get a good education, eat right and get enough sleep, sit up straight and SMILE! You know about most of these. Oy, do you know about these. What I'd like to help with are the ones that we tend to avoid: Like learning how not to be your own worst enemy, and how to face and eliminate your biggest problems These two are often inter-twined.

Being honest with yourself is key. It is always key. A primary part of this (being-honest-with-yourself) stuff involves separating your identity from who your caregivers and supporters think you are, and have tried to mold you into. Becoming yourself, or the person you would like to be, often includes as much *unlearning* as new learning.

The Parent Trap

The power of the parental relationship in shaping your outlook of yourself and your prospects for life goes beyond your parents' overt wishes for you. As progeny, kids naturally feel bound to their parents' destiny. Realizing this pull, you can resist, you can dispassionately see the many unnecessary traps this leads to. You don't have to be like your folks, and you don't have to be the opposite of your folks. Resist the urge to be in narrow comparison with them. You are you. Become your independent self. The more your caregivers allow and encourage this the better. The more they resist, the more likely it is that they are insecure about themselves, and the more cautious you should be about the relationship.

Most of the older folks around you, your parents primarily, often have very strong notions about how you should be, and what you should be working on in terms of improvement. Usually this means their agenda of what they think is best for you, not them support-ively helping you with your (stupid) (unrealistic) hopes and dreams. Sometimes, if you are attempting to fix some physical or emotional hurt inflicted by their actions, they will try to keep you from dealing with that problem, because they know the solution will expose them as complicit. Sometimes you're trying to fix something that was passed down by a parent because the parent could never deal with it him or herself, like parental abuse, different kinds of prejudice, excess drinking or smoking, passive/aggressive tendencies, sexual dysfunction, a kiss up/shit down mentality, or any of a number of other things. Because of many factors like these, most parents' help is of the "You should study hard," "You should work hard," "Make me proud," "Honor thy father," "Don't do anything to hurt your mother" type. Since we live in a country where good parenting skills are about as common as a buffalo sighting, lots of folks have this problem.

I hope you are beginning to see why being honest with yourself is so important, and so difficult. Powerful people in your life often don't want you to be too honest with yourself. Parental fear of expo-sure as culpable for their children's problems is a primary reason their children kid themselves into thinking that their biggest problems aren't that big, avoiding the really tough ones, thinking or hoping they will go away. They won't, and if you push them down and act like they're not there, they will reemerge stronger, and more debilitating than ever, and will probably get played out again with your kids. All the primitive cultures shared a common mythology regarding this: Don't run from your demons, they are with you and of you; you can not hide from them. Face them, allow them, measure them; and defeat them. **You *can* defeat them.** This is the hardest, and best, kind of triumph. The rest will seem easy–er.

This whole section probably seems parentally harsh. It is, but it is not a call for parental rejection. This society encourages an idealization of parents, a false hierarchical view that is pervasive. We defer to parents in all matters relating to their children short of overt and reported abuse. Anyone can gain parental power simply through (an accident of) intercourse. Parents go through no schooling, or on-the-job training, or evaluation, yet are the be-all and end-all for their children. For too many kids this false hierarchical view has been the mantra of their largely dysfunctional lives. I am not encouraging anyone to stop loving his or her parents, but to cut the psychic umbilical cord and to love them as the (flawed) human beings that we are.

Nets

When I was a hip young hippie, like you crazy kids, we had a saying about folks like me: "Never trust anyone over 30." It's a great saying, and mostly true. We know why it's true. People "sell out." Even if they don't, they change. Responsibilities begin. Loans come due. You get a *real* job. Your peers start getting partnered—there's always peer pressure. You get too old to hang out in the clubs, even if you still want to. Babies can be a big factor in this. Your folks make you move out of the house. Even if they don't, eventually it just gets too embarrassing. And these are just the obvious things.

It's the insidious stuff that's the real problem, and it's already started to snag you: Your family's values and loyalties, your religion, ethnicity, socio-economic status, circle of friends, musical tastes, hobbies or sports, high school, college, sorority or fraternity. All of these loyalties that benefit you also exact a certain amount of your independence. As you are about to see, this all happens very innocently.

When you're young your folks begin throwing little nets on you, say by sending you to Sunday School. Next it's Brownies or Cub Scouts and team sports. It's part of the civilization process that all of us (originally) little heathens are put through. Problem is, this is normally done by people with a narrow point of view. Think how different your acculturation would be, how different you might be, if your parents had a narrow Buddhist, or Eskimo, or other point of view. You may have less affinity for their style than some parental-type should-ers think, though that will rarely stop them from imposing this on you. To the contrary, the more different you seem, usually the more effort is expended to make you conform. In the past this had more value. An Eskimo who acted like a Tahitian in the frozen North would encounter some uncommon problems. Today a global marketplace allows and encourages you to find your own bliss. Is there a spot on the map calling you? Check it out! Is there something you've always wanted to try? (This is too easy.) TRY!

By the time you're reading this book, even though you think you're still a free agent, you have a lot of affective nets hung over you. Since you're so used to them you hardly notice, but if you tried to shuck them, to *unlearn* them, your parents, teachers, preachers, and those types would let you know pretty quickly that they were there. So why make trouble? No reason, if you don't mind being sold out by the time you hit, say, 30!

Right about now is your first and last chance to shake off the nets that you aren't sure you want, and learn how to keep shaking, because there are always more. What happens to most folks is the nets keep piling up and tangling up in different ways. By the time you're about 30, 35 if you're really hip, you are caught beyond escape. After that, lots of folks start seeking out nets, they become regular net freaks. Join this, join that. The more exclusive it is, the more they want to join. Exclusive means not only that it's great to be in, but that most other people are kept out. I'm not much of a joiner. I don't much like the idea of joining up with exclusive people. They have this habit of joining together to exclude people for their own narrow benefit. Besides, I start getting tangled up in those damn nets.

Do What **You** Want to Do

Lou Reed wrote a song about a woman named Suzanne. Part of it said,

> *You do what you want to do, and you do it well.*
> *You do what you want to do and I love you Suzanne.*

Simple words, but pretty cool. This little piece of poetry is a good endorsement for doing what *you* want to do with *your* life. If you do what you want to do, it makes you feel good. If you do what you want to do, you do it well, because you're doing what you want to do. And if you do what you want to do, and naturally do it well, some cool person like Lou Reed will love you for it.

The next key to doing what you want to do is having the ability, and paying your dues to acquire all of the skills to be able to be what you want to be. Ability is a tricky thing. How do you know if you have the ability to become a doctor, or an NBA player? Well if you're short, that could limit you in the NBA, but then again there is 5'5" Mugsey Bogues doing just fine in the Land of the Giants. So maybe the best way to see if you can attain some of those long shot dreams is to try them. Realizing that they're long shots, though, means that you don't neglect the rest of your package.

Foundation

Tiger Woods and Tanya Harding are good examples of the importance of developing a well-rounded package. Tiger, even though he was pretty sure he would be able to make some nice money playing golf, kept up with his school work, learned how to communicate well, kept in touch with and interested in the rest of the world. Poor old Tanya was tracked as an idiot-savant figure skater by her parents. Her desperation to be successful at this was fueled by the fact that it was the *only* thing she was good at. She had a very shaky foundation, Tiger has a very strong one. You need a broad, strong foundation.

The right foundation is different for each one of us, but well-formed foundations share many common elements.

It is natural to emphasize your strengths, what comes easy, or more naturally for you, but not so good to do this at the expense of those things that are a struggle for you. A super strong chair leg on one corner can not compensate for a weak one on another corner. For example, if you emphasize those things that will bring you great financial success, while neglecting your personality development, your wealth may not bring you or your family much happiness. Don't cripple yourself with a vulnerable foundation. This goes back to fixing your biggest problems and not being your own worst enemy.

Give your worst subject in school at any time plenty of attention. It is a simple logic, especially during that long period in your life before most of you settle on a clear path. Use this time to eliminate

s in your foundation, weaknesses that may close doors to
 nay ultimately want to do, or weaknesses that will hamper
your ability to find lasting happiness, or to be a good partner, or
parent, or citizen.

This is also the best time to pursue your (long-shot) dreams, to
risk failing at that which you most want, to at least know that you
gave it a shot, and not to forever wonder if you could have made it.

Humility

Few things are more misunderstood in our culture than the value
of humility. It is the approximate opposite of arrogance, but exists
quite nicely in a person along with confidence, competence and success. It stems (in part) from an understanding that each of us is one
of billions of people in this world, most born with tremendous
potential, and all deserving of equal rights, protections and opportunities.

Humility works to minimize hierarchy, recognizing its necessity
in a crowded complex world, while vigilantly guarding against its
abuse. Hierarchical people are constantly caught up in comparisons—their opinions of others often tainted by (perceived) position,

as if the free market *were* magically fair and accurate in its human apportionments, or each person given equal opportunity.

Successful people are more vulnerable to arrogance than others. Success is often corrupting. The successful rationalize that they worked hard, used their considerable potential wisely, and have been properly rewarded. Their position brings them privilege and benefits greater than other people's, reinforcing this impression of superiority. They *have* done better.

Humble people recognize how this can all be accomplished without falling into a trap of superiority; of arrogance. They don't take for granted the innate strengths and cultural advantages that have boosted their chances. They recognize that most people work hard, that the hard-working offspring of an Ivy League family have an artificial leg up on the equally hard-working children of poor third-world peasants, and that if switched at birth, the fortune of success would switch just as surely.

Humility enables ever-greater circles of love and understanding. Witter Bynner, in a most wonderful linguistic discovery, suggested that the origin of the word "understand" was to "stand under." Whatever implications may or may not be drawn from this, it is clear to me that you cannot overstand others, be superior to them, if you would understand them. It is said that before one person can help another person, he or she must find in him or herself what is the matter in the other.   Must *understand* the problem in the other. Becoming a good partner, parent, or citizen requires *under* standing, requires humility. Don't let anyone, no matter how powerful, or beautiful, or persistent, strip from you your humility. Humility is your ability to care, to love, to grow, and to become yourself.

The Bubble

We all live in some kind of narrow reality. Poorer folks live in a reality confined by their lack of money, education and opportunity. More affluent people have a different problem. Though they live with many more options, their normal level of comfort restricts them from viewing much of the other human realities because most are less *comfortable* than theirs. The more comfortable you become, the more difficult it is to accept discomfort as a learning experience. So affluent Americans want to live with other affluent Americans, send their kids to school with kids like theirs, worship with folks like them, belong to clubs, socialize, travel, be with people they are comfortable with. This, then, is what is referred to as "The Bubble."

The Bubble is why rich folks don't understand poorer folks; can allow themselves to think there is something wrong with them; can project anything they want onto them. Here's a little insight on how this bubble thing works. A family with an income of $35,000 per year is in the top 5% of the world's populace, based on income. People living in The Bubble making this kind of money sure don't think of themselves as belonging in the richest 5% of the world's people, but it is financially true.

So who's rich? Living in the bubble is distorting, isn't it?

I have left The Bubble from time to time, though to be honest, less lately as I have become more comfortable. The people outside of it are just fine. Lovely. They are as nice as the people inside, just different. Problem is they are always having to divide a pie with too few pieces in it. It is generally not the fault of these people that this is so, but it is often the fault of the people inside. The people inside never realize this because they never leave. They are just too comfortable.

To become yourself you have to leave The Bubble. Most of Massachusetts, Ohio, Louisiana, California, (your state here), Canada, Australia, Japan, and Europe don't count. Luxury hotels in tropical paradises don't count. Planned tours to natural wonders in the Third World don't count. They are all just extensions of The Bubble. Mountain climbing, whitewater rafting and other adventurings are good character builders for other things, but are no substitute either. Get out there and live in the rest of the world's shoes for awhile. You must see who they are, because they are most of us. The only way to see who you are is to find out who they are. Knowing yourself in the full human context is vital to becoming yourself.

Once you leave The Bubble, you'll finally be able to see The Bubble. It is no sin to be a knowing resident of The Bubble; the shame is in being unknowing, and uncaring.

Slackers

"Slackers" is a moniker hung on this present coming-of-age generation. Slacking is supposed to be some bad thing. You know, "...nose to the grindstone," "Idle hands make idle minds," "the Protestant work ethic," "Make money, make money, make money."

Today my generation is shovelling the same shit on you that we bitched about when our folks shovelled it on us. What you call this hypocrisy is a generational thing. We old folks like to call it "irony" though that's not what we called it when we were young. What do you call it?

Slacking is just fine, in fact, when you're young, you should be slacking, you should be enjoying life. I mean, what the hell is the rush? This is when you feel good, look good, have the fewest responsibilities, and can party a lot without feeling like shit in the morning. It is very likely the time of your lives. Don't let the should-ers ruin it for you just because they either forgot how much fun it was, or may have ruined it for themselves.

You've just spent the last twenty years getting molded into something that you may not want to be, and now everybody wants to rush you into becoming what you may not want to be for the next sixty or seventy years. That is their problem, babe. Everybody wants to lay their trip on you. Misery *does* love company.

This leads to another part of the becoming-your-best-and-most-comfortable-self puzzle. There is no point where you have to completely give up your slacker ways and become perpetually busy. You don't have to get locked into a life that's so busy that you can't keep a perspective on what you're doing. Being too busy all the time is a prime affliction of modern society. It is a very real form of civilized insanity.

We have seen technological breakthrough after breakthrough to reduce the work load and strain of life, and what do we have today: a society of stressed out, multi-phobic workaholics, too frightened to slow down, too bought-in to rock the boat, and too busy to raise their children. If not working hard or shopping hard, they're playing hard, or busy doing somebody else's (their boss's, their parents') idea of the right thing. Gee, and they keep having trouble keeping a family together. No problem, just start a new family and *try harder!*

It's not worth it, and, it's not the only way.

Climb off the treadmill. You don't *need* 57 pairs of shoes. Please stop right here and read again what Mark Twain said in the front of the book. No one has ever said it better, or ever will. There is another way to get more of what you want. Want less, need less, use less; have more. You don't have to trade things for relationship, for love, for caring, or for time.

This is not a call for imbalance in another direction—a contempt for the material, or for the benefits of hard work, diligence and self-discipline. Seek balance, and you will be moving in the right direction. Fixing what is most wrong with you will make you most right. And that's about the best we can do in this here human condition.

"Turn On, Tune In, Drop Out"

"Timothy Leary's dead" was a famous line; from a famous song; by a famous band, The Moody Blues; about a famous guy; in a famous time, the 60s. Most of you have never heard of Timothy Leary. This is as it should be.

Timothy Leary was glorified, like so many of today's notorious people, for doing more harm than good. He told a generation of adolescent aspirers to hip hippiness to take some acid, check out the counterculture, and to quit being the company's straw boss/dog.

Psychedelia

The "Turn On" part had the biggest downside.

Most folks enjoyed psychedelic drugs at first, many had "doors of perception" opened, and a lot had a great time, finally totally free of the bindings of convention and someone else's idea of duty. But there were problems. Acid didn't come with any directions or warning labels, which is something like giving someone a fancy gun and not telling them where the bullets come out. All bootlegged shit, it was often just that—mind-fucking unpredictable shit. The L.A. Free Press used to print a monthly free mail-in drug analysis in the early seventies. It was a rare occasion if the acid, mescaline, or THC sent in was the real deal; usually it was PCP and some combination of speed, or strychnine.

I remember once splitting two caps of what was sold to us as Woodrose seeds with three friends and then heading off for some boardwalk fun. Woodrose is a Hawaiian hallucinogen similar in its effect to peyote. Two of the folks split one cap, one started nodding and the other turned speed freak, but nothing psychedelic. My cap partner also turned speedy but nothing much happened to me until much later when, on the way home on my bike, I started losing my vision. I barely made it home before I lost it all. I groped my way up the stairs, got shit scared, and bummed half the night before finally falling asleep, with the faint hope that I could see in the morning, so I could hunt the motherfucker down that did this to me.

During the subsequent melodramatic shakedown it came out that the dirty dealer had just taken all his leftover powdered shit, mixed it up, and marketed it as Woodrose. Hence two speeders, a down freak and one "Uh, sorry about the temporary blindness thing, man."

Happy endings are great, but a lot of people weren't so lucky. Some folks committed suicide, accidentally in a hallucinogenic confusion, or purposefully in a hallucinogenic fantasy. Acid occasionally brought on schizophrenia—sometimes temporary, sometimes permanent. A good friend of ours has been trying to walk off too many bad trips on the county's roads for the past twenty-five years now. For a very few, occasionally tripping over the years has been a fairly safe and poignant reminder that helps them keep a perspective on their place in the cosmos. Ultimately most folks couldn't handle it because A) they grew up in some distorted bubble of reality B) their biochemistry was not ideally suited to the drug or C) acid, whether pure, or in some bootlegged concoction, was often just too powerful and unpredictable.

My sources tell me that in today's new generation designer drug marketplace things are much the same. That shortcuts to Ecstasy are the same shortcuts to Hell. Speed still rots your teeth, coke is still a fast train to nowhere, angel dust is still made from large animal tranquilizer, and acid is no more likely "safe" than 25 years ago.

So, there's your warning label: Caveat emptor, Your Hip Highnesses!

"What Is Hip?"

"Tune-in" had less risk, but the whole counterculture thing became too much of an "Us" versus "Them" thing on both sides. The idea was good though, and still is. Get out of your rut. Move from mono to stereo. Check out the flip side of things.

If you're a nerd, explore ways to be physical, to check out the darker side. Take some chances. Dare to "just say 'no'" to your parents, teachers and linear career paths. Don't allow yourself to be pruned to death by all the paranoid empirical "should-ers" yearning for the validity of your allegiance.

Are you a juicer and/or druggie? Clean up! Cut your losses, dudes and dudettes. Don't drink if you wind up in the bottle, don't do dope if the dope does you. Do the right thing. Get some discipline in your life. Get help if you need it. It's OK to admit you have a problem and are weak.

We all have problems and we're all weak in different ways, mostly we just hide it well in this jive-assed human charade where *we all think everyone else is strong while we know we can't show that we are weak*. This is such a significant aspect of human nature. Everybody at the party is *acting* cool and thinking, "Man, look at all these cool people." Meanwhile, everybody's afraid to open up to one another because everybody else looks way too cool for them; but coolness—aloofness—is usually just a mask for insecurity.

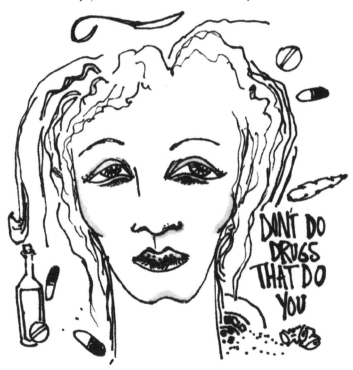

People with addictive personalities have been damaged by others, so they, especially, want to hide the injury, affect a mask. If you need a mask, you probably need help. It takes courage to take off the mask. It takes courage to look, and ask, for help. With courage, many wonderful things become possible.

Were you brought up in some fundamentalist religion, were you instructed to have blind faith in a dogma that does not exist except in the constructs of its own superstitions? Take off the sunglasses, throw away the cane. Explore religious freedom. Hey, it's your right, says so right in the Constitution. (And tell me about this oxymoronic logic of religious fundamentalists of all stripes who are against abortion as robbing a fetus of the constitutional right to life, liberty and the pursuit of happiness, but deny their own children freedom of religion by brainwashing them with a single myopic dogma from the beginning of life, perpetuating a cycle of prejudice and paranoia, a key ingredient in the potion that continues to poison humanity.)

Are you straight? Understand the homosexual. They aren't the norm, but they are as normal as you or me.
Are you white? Learn about the experiences of non-whites.

Are you privileged? Study the humanity of as many of those as you can in the multitude of human misfortune.

Thinking you are better than "others" is the beginning of permanent distortion. Hold that thought, then you'll begin to be 'tuned-in.'

Unreal Expectations

"Drop out" is the last part of Leary's brilliant riff, and damn near as damaging as the first part. Let's try to suck what's good out of this too, before we put the whole weird thing back in the time crapper where it belongs.

We were supposed to drop out of "THE SYSTEM," but the damn "SYSTEM" was what grew the food, built the houses, kept our sorry asses warm in the winter time, gave us the bread to get high, look cool, and buy Dead albums. So the "drop out" part made a few people colder than hell for awhile, and forced most of the rest into a hypocrisy that eventually led back into the "System's" suck-your-spirit-out womb.

"Drop out" got confused too often with "Don't sell out." Having contact with any part of the system made you a traitor. It was like, "Don't breath that polluted air, man. You'll be selling out, man."

Creating unreal expectations begets failure. "The System" is all that there is, folks, unless you are ready to check out. The real game is to get what you want out of the system without being sucked in by it. If you get too greedy it's probably gonna get you. It just kind of starts sticking to you like gooey shit. Leaves a little smell on you too. Lots of times you can even see it, you start smelling so bad.

My all-time hero at this was Mikhail Gorbachev. Old Gorby came up through the commie ranks as an A-1 company man. I'm sure he did some dirty shit, had to as head of the KGB for a while, but all the time he kept his eye on the prize, and when he got to the top he started pulling the plug on all this totalitarian shit. So hooray for Gorby, but for everyone like him there are a million who got sucked in and turned weasely in their soft "go-along, get-along" easy chair. So be careful dancin with the Man too much, you may forget your own tune.

60/40

We feel the hurts inflicted on ourselves more than the hurts we inflict on others; we tend to see 50/50 give and take as a 60/40 proposition. The simple example is physical pain. Stick a pin in your hand, then in someone else's hand. Discounting any reaction to this by the other person, which hurt more?

This is a primary way that two individuals can each feel wronged or shortchanged by the other.

This is a primary way groups feel self-righteously wronged or insulted by each other.

It is a primary cause for individual, group, ethnic, religious, national, you-name-it-we-got-it human conflict.

Give the other person/group the benefit of the doubt without thinking that you've done them a favor. You probably haven't. You'll just be balancing out your predilection to see 50/50 as 60/40.

Capitalism

Capitalism is the most talked about and written about subject there is. It is a huge part of human existence. It is The System. Having some understanding of The System is good personal business, it is personally profitable, and, like it or not, it is real important to understanding life here in Babylon.

Lots of coming-of-agers, myself—once upon a time—included, make the mistake of blaming the entire System for its flaws. This is unfortunate, and a waste of time. It is the only game in town, and fortunately for humanity, it is the best *economic* system so far imagined. If we could just come up with a political system to complement and balance it—say, democracy—we'd really be in business. [See "Politics," page 119.]

The System has many levels. Most of us operate at the primary worker/consumer level, and most of us have a fair idea how this part works: You make some money, pay too much of it in taxes, spend most of the rest on what you need, blow what's left, and then make some more. Meanwhile, you're mostly concerned with your life and the lives of the people who are close to you. In our daily existence The System generally affects us in pretty mundane and manageable ways. Things change dramatically as we climb the ladder into the rarefied air of high finance, and though we have few dealings with this environment, it is very important to our well-being. Let's take a look at the higher levels for a while.

Mega Money

Philosophy, morality, or anything else for that matter, usually becomes subordinate when you start talking about big money—and that is as it should be. In high finance everything is strictly business. Profit and Loss are the higher gods. This is why it is necessary for some to have an in-depth involvement in the financial world and its many big-monied parts. In a world as incredibly rich and intricate as ours, it is very important for lots of people to do this work, and to become very wealthy in the process, even amassing huge personal fortunes. Even the most optimal and humane capitalism creates great wealth. The money is out there, and if all the good folks are content to shuffle by and concentrate on smelling the roses, sure as hell some megalomaniac will come along, make and take all that money, and maybe start charging for rose smellin. So don't knock the rich folks too hard. Their wealth and retention of *small* blocks of power is very stabilizing.

The rules of the System's big money game are simple: Win any way you can. If you don't understand that going in, you will quickly become, like any novice in a savvy poker game, an appetizer. Some of the results of this game make the St. Valentine's Day Massacre, and other underworld high jinks, look like a child's game of jacks. The game needs really strong referees. That's been one of the big problems with the System—everybody, looking for any edge they can get, constantly buying off the referees.

"Power is corrupting" is one of the **Great Truths**, right up there with "Flat flip flies straight." Power is certainly a head trip. It is why few who play the game are able to maintain a firm grip on their humanity and humility. Whether power emanates from fortune, fame, position, or some combination thereof, it can rival any drug in addictive compulsion. That is why free and open markets that maximize this diffusion of power are one of humanity's best protections against super-powerful super-assholes. So, it's actually good to have lots of rich folks. We just have to find better ways to keep their power confined to economic matters, to keep them equal in the eyes of the law and in our electoral process, and to make entry into the financial elites as fair as possible. These are old problems. Each new solution initiates new attempts at circumvention, because the primary goals of wealthy capitalists are to maintain selfish advantage, and to gain greater wealth.

Capitalism and You: Imperfect Together

Capitalism is all the rage these days. Communism is terminal. We won. The stock market is going berserko. Capitalism's future is rosy, its potential seemingly limitless. Remote foreign places are less often referred to as "impoverished third-world countries" or as "potential hot spots," and much more as "emerging markets." The invisible hand is reaching out and touching everybody and everything, everywhere.

I could write a long polemic on the wonders of capitalism: creating jobs, a higher standard of living, the promise of freedom, and long-denied political empowerment. I could also write persuasively of exploitation of the masses for the wealth of a few, of the dumping of high-paying American jobs overseas, of exporting the lowest common denominators of our culture for a fast buck—like how the now-deported Joe Camel is cruising the rest of the globe creating 12-year-old nicotine addicts. This is all very important stuff, but I will spare us.

More important to you is how **you** deal with capitalism. For advice, the best place to go is to the source. Adam Smith is the Big Mac Daddy of capitalism. Though a lot of bottom-line social Darwinists have used his name in vain to rationalize their views, old Adam was a pretty thoughtful and cool dude. Over two hundred years ago he had a line on these types, and rejected their view of capitalism.

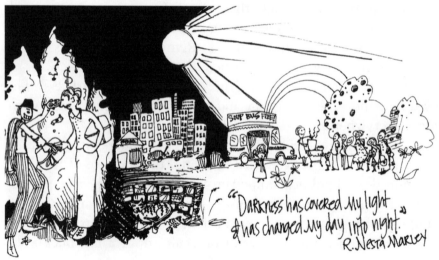

"Darkness has covered my light & has changed my day into night."
R. Nesta Marley

Society may subsist among different men,
as among different merchants, from a sense of
utility, without any mutual love or affection, and
though no man in it should owe any obligation,
or be bound in graditude (sic) to any other, it may
still be upheld by a mercenary exchange of good
offices according to an agreed valuation.

Adam understood how capitalism elevated to too lofty a position
could be damaging, how the "money fever" distorts cooperation and
mutual respect, and he knew how to keep commerce in proportion
to all of the other attributes of successful community.

All members of a human society stand in
need of each other's assistance, and are likewise
exposed to mutual injuries. Where the necessary
assistance is reciprocally afforded from love, from
graditude (sic), from friendship and esteem, the
society flourishes and is happy. All the different
members of it are bound together by the agreeable
bands of love and affection, and are, as it were,
drawn to one common centre of mutual good offices.

Now that's capitalism. Working together, looking out for one another, cooperating. Cooperation is not always easy. It is often complicated and difficult; but it is always easier, and better, than the alternatives.

> When people work together,
>   There is a profit to share.
> When people work apart,
>   They sacrifice the sharing.
> When people work against one another,
>   There is a harvest of thorns.

Love & Sex

In Search of Emotional & Sexual Happiness

My views are about heterosexual love because I am heterosexual.

At its best, the most pleasurable thing in the world is to make love with a partner of mutual love and affection.

A woman is most content when her lover lingeringly and regularly pleasures her to satisfaction out of a bond of love and respect.

A man is most content when he knows that the woman he loves, loves him and finds him sexually satisfying.

This can be our own little piece of heaven, something we can hold in the pocket of our souls as we muddle our way through the rest of an often difficult life.

So, why do we spend so little time in heaven?

Let's get the sorry sordid history of all this out of the way, so we can get to fixing things up.

First, in true All-American fashion, let's blame somebody.

The Limp Prick as Cultural Icon

It is a profound wonder of the world how civilization has managed to come this far protecting the fragile male ego against thousands of years of contrary evidence. Erica Jong etched her name atop the pantheon of whistle blowers when she posed that if men weren't so inadequate in bed they wouldn't have had to spend so much of the rest of their time trying to prove women inadequate in other places. Her famous image is of the "limp male prick" faced with a woman's "wonderful all-weather cunt" that "neither storm, nor sleet, nor dark of night could faze." "It was always there, it was always ready. No wonder men hated women. No wonder they invented the myth of female inadequacy."

Five thousand years of the empirical wisdom of western civilization felled by a single stinging paragraph...

Of course men had to build empires, go to war, and construct huge monuments attesting to their greatness. Hell, when things got a little shaky, they even deified a few of the boys: Buddha, Jesus, Mohammed, all very possibly because men couldn't get it done in the sack.

Were the reverse true, we might all still be walking around in

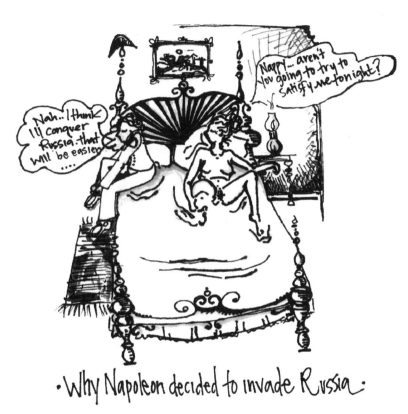

· Why Napoleon decided to invade Russia ·

(easily accessible) loincloths, eating nuts and berries, wandering around with stupid grins on our faces.

It may be an exaggeration to say that guns, tanks, rockets and atomic bombs are mere pyrotechnic proof of men's poor penile performance. Or that Euclidean geometry, Newtonian physics and Pythagorean poppycock were all high intellectual masturbation for the proof that couldn't be found in our pudding. It would certainly not be inaccurate to say that fancy motorcycles, cars, and boats are more often phallic frauds proclaiming an absence of real talent.

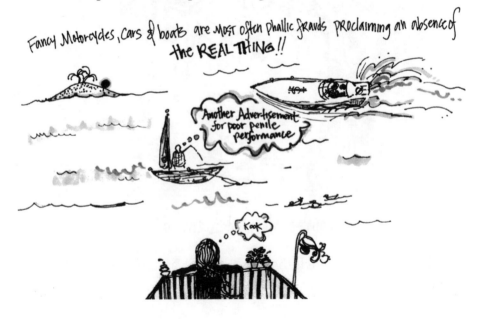

And women's first priorities aren't diamonds and furs, though they are smart enough to take them if that's the best their men can do. What women want is love, sweet love, and SATISFACTION!

So what's the problem with the guys?

The problem is it's not EASY. It can't be done by just squeezing a trigger or puffing out a chest. The ability to walk erect and to think abstractly are often cited as separating man from less intelligent life. But where, oh where, is that wonderful awareness of the potential to profoundly pleasure his mate. Unfortunately, throughout HIStory, few men have found enough interest in her story.

Diamonds are ok —
if that's the best a man
can do — but a woman wants
the real thing.. Love sweet love.

39

Shopping to Fill the Void

As most sociological phenomena are double-edged swords, male sexual inadequacy does have an upside. It creates a primal force for our consumerist society. Many women, constantly sexually under-nourished, have an insatiable desire to fill their unmet needs, and attempt to do this by **consuming** everything in sight. Their brave men, facing their inadequacies in the bedroom, work to (dis)prove (the absence of) their manhood by pillaging and plundering to feed their mates' voracious appetites.

I suspect that this is the reason the fashion magazines are in cabal to print inane or counterproductive articles about love and sex. Accurate information would begin a chain reaction leading to reduced advertising revenue and interest in these rags in the first place. Articles like "Make Your Man Want You More!" and "Light His Fire With Lingerie" only shorten the time between a woman's last tryst with her lover and her next shopping spree.

Let's go over the problem again and see if, after 5000 *odd* years, we can take a small step toward a happier ending.

Men's physical needs are easily met with an ejaculation. This is so easily done that usually all a man needs is a picture of a woman, a lubricant, and a few minutes alone. Men's spiritual needs are quite different. In order to satisfy these, a woman must display great pleasure and satisfaction in the love act. The mere act of masturbation, either with or without a woman, is not spiritually sustaining, and without a woman's show of appreciation (real or feigned), will not bring peace of mind.

Without peace of mind, the stud becomes aggressive; he must fill his own void. This is done in many ways. The most aggressive choose some type of combat, but usually it is accomplished by watching others in a gladiator competition while consuming alcohol until reaching a merciful stupor.

Women are different. (Thank you Jesus, thank you Lord!) They are not so easily satisfied physically, or spiritually for that matter. In fact it is very helpful if a synthesis of the two is offered. Like it or not, women generally want the real thing.

Male Mea Culpa

Things get a little tricky here, and I'd like to take a moment to provide a little background before continuing with my line of thinking.

Though I've made the case for laying this state of affairs at the feet of men generally and historically, it is not fair to place too much of the blame on any one man. Most of us try to do the best we can with what we've got and what we know; unfortunately the latter is usually no more adequate than the former.

Some of these things are not so clear-cut and obvious absent thorough overview, so in the interest of a male mea culpa, I will offer a defense, or at least some reasonable excuses.

First, men, by nature of testosterone, are competitive, especially when it comes to winning a mate. Let's face it ladies, there is a direct DNA link between us and those rams you always see butting heads on "Nature." The point being that if a guy has some useful insight on pleasuring his woman, he sure as hell isn't going to take out an ad in the local paper.

Next, some women send out mixed messages. (Shocking, isn't it?!) This is mostly because, although women generally know what they want, they're often not sure who they want it from. Younger women are more susceptible to this. They don't know who they want because they have little experience in these matters, because so much of the information given to them is conflicted, and because when you're fifteen and horny, lots of guys look good. Since this is a young man's first exposure to the mating game, it's no wonder we start out confused.

As if things weren't bad enough, guys try to impress the objects of their affection in almost all the wrong ways because we try to impress them with the things that impress us, not them. "I hunt, I compete, I own, I win, Ayayay!"

Many young ladies, moving from one dashed romantic possibility to another, develop their own new set of misconceptions. Toss in a little poor parenting, and other types of childhood abuse, and this ongoing sad situation makes a lot more sense.

So it's a mess, and a mess that's really not anybody's fault.

Repairing the Stud

Getting out of this vicious cycle individually really isn't that difficult though. For guys with a mind of their own, who can really see what's in their, and their partner's, and ultimately everyone else's best interest, the solution is easy to see, if not necessarily easy to accomplish. It starts by recognizing two simple facts: Women take longer to satisfy sexually, and women find satisfaction in differing ways than men. These two ideas, merged, provide the best framework for success.

The first leads to the need for a man to learn to control his ejaculation. There are two primary ways to accomplish this. The first is to simply to wait until you get old and your plumbing starts to go. The better way is to read about the many known techniques of ejaculation control, and practicing the ones that seem best suited for you.

The second is recognizing that your partner often appreciates different things, and is stimulated at different times and in different ways, than you. It took me a long time to realize that my girlfriends really didn't want to watch me play ball, or care if I could catch a peanut with my mouth, or how far I could stick my tongue down their throat, or how fast I could make my prick move. Figuring out what your lover wants is not the easiest thing to do, but seeing what you want and then projecting it on her is a sure recipe for failure. Listen to her. It's OK to ask her. This is a start in the right direction, and although it's just a start, it sure as hell beats macho marching off in the wrong direction. I always liked that quote that said "A boy can make a baby. It takes a man to be a father." The same idea is aptly applied to being a good lover.

All men have experienced ejaculation without satisfying their mates. It is the sad norm, it is what this essay seeks to address. The beautiful, magnificent woman you were just making passionate love with has, upon completion of your ejaculation, just turned into an unattractive and insatiable pest who won't let you sleep, and who wants you, can you believe it, to hold her and cuddle her. Who would prefer this to a beautiful woman satisfied in your arms, and you still loving, ready, and eager to please her again and again?

What we're talking about here is emphasizing a woman's satisfaction as the man's best satisfaction. The peak experience, believe it or not guys, is to deeply satisfy your mate while refraining from having an orgasm. The man gets to bask in the joy of his woman's satisfaction, while maintaining his ability to perform again and again.

Who could have more wealth than this?

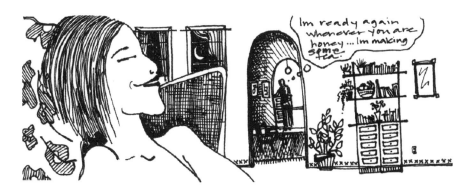

Emotionally and sexually satisfying relationships come in all shapes and sizes. They are interwoven with many overlaid circumstances, in each instance creating their own unique and wonderful union. Physical attraction is important, but sustaining attraction and keeping it healthy, nurturing, and mutually respectful requires achieving comfort levels across a whole spectrum of criteria. How quickly love can fade in the face of selfishness, sloth, infidelity, or simply letting yourself go.

When it comes to relationships, the best motto may be, "Life is a matter of what have you done for me lately." Being caring last year, or even last week, is not very sustaining to a partner who wants and needs your support today.

Marriage

Marriage is a scary subject for young adults. Rightly so. The up and down sides to it have such long lasting reverberations. That is why a take-your-time process, with lots of practice, is best. There can be exceptions to this rule, like any others, but as the world continues to complicate, it becomes more and more important.

Practice, practice, practice. Dating, relationships, and living together, if done with the care and effort that any partner deserves, are invaluable tools for later marital success. It takes practice to be good at anything. Why would anyone want to jump into a lifelong commitment to another without lots of practice?

You are practicing, however, with another human being. Their feelings are, at least temporarily, entrusted to you. Learning and displaying mutual caring, sharing and respect is what you are practicing. It is also extremely important to **practice safely.** You are practicing a real life game. The consequences are real. This practice time is also when you get to see what problems from your past may be getting in the way of a successful future.

A good marriage is the bomb. There is nothing better. It is the fundamental, most important, most natural union of cooperation in this life. I'm not talking about some old strictly-hetero, gotta-have-the-perfect-wedding, do-your-duty, have-(screwed-up)-kids, gotta-go-to-church, hide-the-dysfunction, as-long-as-we-look-good, bullshit marriage. I'm talking about a romantic life journey shared between two loving adults. Something that doesn't start going downhill a day, or a year, after it begins.

If worked at, a good marriage will grow ever more beautiful year after year. There is a **real magic** that grows from the deep sharing of love, sexuality, nurturing, and experience. It creates something way bigger than the whole of its parts. There are so many things a good partner is in a marriage: friend, lover, supporter, sidekick, leader, follower, protector, and able shit detector (in cases when the other partner's gets temporarily clogged).

Kids are a whole other thing. There's just too much to talk about. The best start to good parenting, though, is good partnering that resulted from two people who individually got their own shit together.

Finding a Partner

The J. Geils Band had a great song a long time ago called "Love Stinks." The theme of this song may be the main reason that most of us old folks wouldn't roll back the clock even if we could. The song went something like, "You love her, she loves him, he loves somebody else, you just can't win. Love stinks, yeah, yeah." It is **hard** out there trying to find Mr. or Ms. Right-for-You.

There is no formula for finding the right person. If you attempt to follow artificial criteria, you're likely to screw up your own natural process. Some people get lucky early. Some that think they got lucky early soon find out they got (permanently) unlucky early. Sometimes it is a long wait. My favorite aunt, Aunt Clara, didn't find true love until into her late seventies, though she never stopped looking. My wife and I were in our forties before we could find one another. Please don't give up on romantic love. It is the best thing we have. It beats even God, or cats—by a lot.

One last thought on finding the right person. Get your best idea of what that person is looking for, and, "within your own parameters," try to become that person. The best way to find the right person is to become the right person.

The last word is reserved for Queen Erica.

> *"Do you want me to tell you something really subversive?*
> *Love is everything it's cracked up to be."*

Religion

The fundamental problem of traditional religion has been the human need to embellish. In all the modern religions, the need to deify a human being began the first twist in truth's path, and, once the compass heading of the truth is lost, "white can appear black, enough a lack."

And so in the Biblical story of the loaves and fishes, the simple reward of sharing becomes the alchemy of a miracle. Moses must accomplish a litany of superhuman feats to legitimize ten commandments of simple integrity. I'm no theologian but the other great religions all share the same "our God is better than your God" hyperbole. The Buddha sat under the bonsai tree so long it turned into a rock. The prophet Mohammed wrote the entire Koran without getting up to take a leak or anything.

I still think we in the Judeo-Christian thing win the pissing contest. Moses parted the Red Sea, and Jesus arose from the dead after three days (with no brain damage or anything), forgave and offered groovy life everlasting to all who pledged allegiance.

"Beat that Allah!"

"What you say?"

"I'll kick your turbaned ass cause my God's better than your god any day."

And so it goes. Disagree about Jesus with a lot of folks around here and you risk a punch in the nose, or worse. Head over to the Middle East and question the holiness of Allah and you'll be in even deeper shit. Stop by Tel Aviv and question the miracles of Moses and a whole other world of indignation will probably come down on you. Meanwhile, at their conservative cores, fundamentalists burn with self-righteous hatred for one another. It doesn't end there. Hindus, Sikhs, Muslims, and Sufis in southern Asia, warring sects like the Sunni and Shiites in Iraq, and Catholics and Protestants in Northern Ireland all regularly brutalize one another. There are many more, but at least we have taken a good scratch at the surface. "I will kick your ass." "I will rip you limb from limb." "I will happily and gloriously kill your women and babies, in the name of my religion."

It makes you wonder, doesn't it? Makes you wonder how humanity can be so brutally stupid.

It took a lot of practice.

All religions, at their daily human level, are essentially the same.

They all preach love, tolerance, fidelity, and forgiveness. So why do they portray themselves as so different and at odds with one another? Why do religions invoke the supernatural to legitimize the value of the commonly understood?

Natural Devo-lution

The answers are thousands of years old.

Historically, religion and governance have been the twin pillars of *civilized control*. Civil and moral authority have always gone hand in hand. Civil authority needs a moral authority to legitimize it; and a moral authority, at least in the old world order, needed a big army to keep it from being somebody's lunch. Hence, a marriage made on earth, purportedly about heaven.

In the thousands of years *before* the first large civilizations came into being, human cooperation had evolved into organized clans, communities and loose federations of large groups of people. On the local level, folks had learned to get along with one another pretty well, learned the benefits of cooperation versus confrontation, and, except for your basic barbarities, things could be pretty cool. Life was sometimes brutal, but it was certainly natural living.

Culture, too, was a local phenomenon, and religion was a strong part of each local culture for the same reason then as today: human curiosity. "Why are we here?" "What is the purpose of our existence?" and, if you lived in California, "Why is the ground shaking?" Quite naturally, they looked for their answers in their visible surroundings. For obvious reasons the sun, the moon, the earth, fire, water, and wind became prime objects of worship.

As larger civilizations began to form, control of disparate groups brought together under a single governance had to be accomplished. Civil authority's primary tool was a larger, better prepared army that could conquer smaller defenders. The need then was for these smaller groups to come into allegiance with the conquerors, and to not quarrel amongst one another over (cultural) differences.

The easiest thing to do was to take a little of the mythology of each group, and elevate the new combination into something intellectually superior to their old model. There was no need for great sophistication, these people were quite simple. Grandiosity was usually more than sufficient. The bigger the myth (there's nothing much bigger than death and resurrection) and the bigger the physical evidence (See Egypt: the Pyramids), the more easily people yielded their more "primitive" beliefs.

As each new civilization arose, a new, grand, and (not coincidentally) perfectly applicable religion grew within it. The myth of the death and the resurrection wasn't originated in Christianity; it had had a long prior history in smaller venues, but it was raised to its highest art form by the Romans.

"Holy" Shit

The Roman emperors had the same needs as other heads of civilizations, and it is no coincidence that it took hundreds of years after the death of Christ for the myth to be properly tailored as the official religion of the (Holy) Roman Empire. You need a long gestation period for a good religion, that was one of the big rubs when it was being considered. A religion, to be taken seriously, has to seem old when you adopt it. It needs a history, to have stood a test of time. Next, and equally important, if the basis of the religion is some impossible superhuman feat, the passing of all eye witnesses and their immediate offspring is essential. Finally, things of this magnitude cannot be done ham-handedly. It was a long running and delicate dance and negotiation between Christian leaders and the minions of the Roman Empire that ultimately led to the marriage of this religion to that state.

The Christian example of the evolution of religion is the one we are most familiar with here in God Bless America, but its parallels elsewhere are well documented. Islam, Hinduism, and Buddhism arose along side of, were assimilated into, and provided moral authority for other great civilizations. As a result, wherever you go in the world, you will encounter religious parochialism. It is, and has been, inevitable.

Blind Faith as Guiding Light

Today, enlightened people not indoctrinated from birth can readily understand the cultural origins of these ornate legends, and the fragile reasoning supporting these narrow views of religion. There are others of high intelligence, and possessing a strong awareness of life's complexities, that still cling to their familiar old myths. Myths of aboriginal origin, later tailored to help control primitive peoples, still hold strong sway today. Over two thousand years of tradition, loyalty, and momentum are not easily dislodged by science, history, or reason.

Nor do I propose trying to dislodge them. There is a difference between proselytizing—trying to convert—and promoting a different, considered to be more rational, point of view. It is possible that "God" appeared in one of these civilizations and that "His" earthly messenger did just what that particular source book said "He" did. It is also possible that "God" was involved in all of these "Histories," and that they are all true. More likely is that the power of these myths has great and lasting attraction to individuals in their lives, especially those who have been raised from birth to believe.

It is, however, very unlikely that "God," any god worthy of our support, would think any less of a person for honestly believing in something else. If there is a benevolent god in this cosmos, its, her, or his message would be accepting and loving of ALL.

Contrasts & Comparisons:

Gaining Insight, Losing Insecurities & Conceits

Too often, we tend to measure ourselves and others in narrow contrast. We get bogged down in comparisons like "She's so thin, so I must be fat," or deciding someone else is great, or a jerk, based on one encounter, character trait, outfit of the day, or a tune that they like—constantly judging other people by very limited, often distorted criteria. It's such a tempting thing, and, it's so **easy.**

Most of these contrasts are often described as being at opposite ends of a line. For instance, young to old is a clearly linear thing, as is short to tall. Other spectrums of contrast are less easily defined, like comparing haves to have-nots. Who's to say what values are more important? How do you cross-measure love vs. health, wealth and security; deprivation vs. disability, or oppression?

The list of human contrast is near endless in possible combination. However, your position in some is much more important to you than in others. Like, for example, the more polar "Are you a boy, or are you a girl?" or the phases Dead and Alive.

Some of the others that we more regularly measure ourselves by are rich/poor, black/white, skinny/fat, smart/dumb, handsome or beautiful/ugly, egocentric/neurotic, athletic/uncoordinated, graceful/clumsy, hip/nerdistic, generous/selfish, honest/lying cheating rat

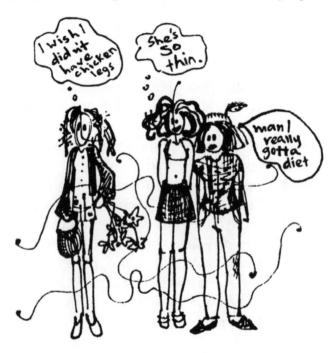

bastard, tough/weak, sensitive/stoic, believing in our god/ally of the devil, etc./etc., etc.

I'm going to offer some observations on some of these contrasts in the hope of broadening your point of view. (More on P.O.V. later.)

White to Black

Might as well get right to it. No matter how much things change, for some reason, this one is still always right at the top of the human comparison heap here in the US of A.

One of the toughest things for me to figure out as a kid was the hierarchy of humanity's ethnic tree. It was always in flux—depending on the criteria, and the mood of the old folks, mostly my old folks, that were doing the judging at any particular time—but mostly it fell within well-traveled limits. What was difficult to understand were the convoluted inconsistencies of the grown-ups. I believe that most kids of my generation—the 50s— shared a general understanding of this ranking, and an awareness that it was mostly crapola. Today there are more differing views on this, but most families still keep their own markers on who's hot and who's not on the human totem pole. Though the old Anglo-Germanic-

Italian-Irish-Jewish-Asian-Latino-Black pecking order is now complicated by gender, sexuality, and moral issues, a constant is that whites are still on top, Blacks still relegated to the bottom.

Another constant is that Blacks are still blamed for their position. They are still stuck in the same Catch 22 they have always been caught in: Other folks avoid them, don't want to live near them, work with them, or associate with them, yet they are supposed to get a job, and fit in. A few Blacks may be okay, the rationale goes, but after that the neighborhood, or classroom, or workplace quickly goes to hell. So what the hell are the others who are left out supposed to do?

Other ethnic minorities that have assimilated into the American melting pot all point with pride to their blue collar roots, and how they lifted themselves up, worked hard and saved, sent their kids to college, and realized the American dream. Now they blame some Blacks for not doing the same.

What many of these proud ethnics conveniently overlook is that they originally got those steady blue collar jobs because Anglos felt it was better to have an Italian mixing cement and laying bricks, that it was better to have a hated Irishman pounding the beat, to have a Jew making their clothes, to have a Polack on the assembly line, or to have a Chinaman building their railroads. Anyone was better than the Black. As the last ones hired and the first ones fired, it was kind of hard to keep a steady job. As the last group accepted into a school, club, or association, it was hard to gain the education, learn the social skills and make the contacts that led to a better life, and, when they did attain them, they were more likely to be called "uppity niggers" than to be offered a better job.

When I was in my late twenties I lived for a time in Argentina. It was a wonderful experience to live in a culture where talk of the U.S. was almost as rare as conversations here are about Argentina. I was often struck by the incredible similarities between people of different cultures and ethnicities who played a similar role in each culture. I kept seeing the same soap operas and similar characters there that I had known here. My wife tells me that I learned what psychologists have known for a long time, that there is more difference among people within an ethnic group than between ethnic groups.

This is far from the whole of it, but it's a real piece. Find out about some more. Holding on to our own insecurities and conceits through narrow comparison plays a crucial part in the continued human tragedy of prejudice. We can't keep blaming folks for not being "in" if we won't let them "in."

Smart/Dumb

What are we measuring? Book smarts? What for? There is lit-tle correlation between academic excellence and financial success, artistic success, having a happy marriage, raising well-adjusted chil-dren, being a good citizen, a good soldier, or a good worker. Hell, this one's too easy. Let's move to the other end.

What's dumb?

Not book smart? I just showed you how much that counted for. Sometimes a person seems dumb, or is just not very good at small talk, or at whatever you happen to be doing when you are with them. I know a man who, through many interactions, I thought of as borderline mentally retarded, only to later find he had a Ph.D. in engineering. He sure as hell was smart at something. Maybe a per-son who seems dumb has a mental disability. How smart would you be if, say, somebody blew out 20% of your circuitry? Would you want someone to devalue you, or someone you cared for, because of a disability beyond your or their control?

Athletic/Uncoordinated and Hip/Nerdistic

Almost everybody envies the graceful athlete and the in-crowd dudes and dudettes, but having had the benefit of too many high school reunions, I know that hipness and athleticism are usually faded flowers by 40. The uncoordinated nerd & nerdette have good knees, a decent life, and, sometimes by just being late bloomers and by not partying too much, often look a helluva lot better.

Besides, we can't all be Al & Peg Bundy.

Tough And Weak

This is one the Gen Xers have done great with. You folks, better than any group to come through yet, have shucked machismo as the crap that it is. It is nice to see, in some ways at least, that evolution is working.

The meanings of tough and weak are evolutionary in the course of an individual life also. Being tough when you're ten may mean screwing up your courage to punch somebody bigger than you in the nose, or defending an unpopular kid unfairly picked on. When you're 30 and starting a family it may mean walking away from a fight and looking like a coward. When you're sixty it may mean, that after working hard all your life and becoming a big success, you are willing to be nursemaid to your elderly parents.

Weakness is another thing. It is insidious in this life. I have always harped on my kids, "Do the right thing," "Do the right thing," "Do the right thing," because things done poorly today easily begin piling up into a compounded mess of a life. A Pepsi and a Twinkie won't make you fat, a smoke or two at a party won't give you lung cancer. Experimenting with different lovers can be a good thing to do when you're young, but can create a devastating trail of wreckage if not grown out of.

Being honest with yourself about what is just a treat and what is becoming a compulsion, or what is good fun and what is hurtful, is vital to successful living. One of the toughest things to do in this life is to be honest with yourself. We are **all** susceptible to denial. One of my favorite sayings is about swimming in "de river of de Nial."

Show how tough you are. Stay out of the river.

Egocentrics & Neurotics

This is a really interesting spectrum of contrast, one that affects us much more than we generally realize. Let's take a look at the egocentric and neurotic *extremes* in this continuum with a little sharper eye on the egocentric, who has historically gotten a far easier ride.

Untempered egocentrics have been the bane of humanity since the Neanderthal man clubbed his way to fame. History's heavies are preponderantly egocentric: Attila the Hun, Leona Helmsley, Adolf Hitler ("after he went too far") and Marge Schott come to mind. I'm sure you have your own Who's Who of villainy, most of whom will likely be egocentric. It is the more garden variety egocentrics, though, that affect us day to day, many that are so close to us that we don't even recognize them as so.

(Listen you neurotics, don't *worry*, I'll get to your problems soon enough.)

Egocentrics are not hard to recognize. They tend to blame the world for their problems and take credit for anything good that happens. Egocentrics are usually bullies with a kiss up/shit down mentality. They're always having to "lay down the law," or "straighten someone out." They are controlling, often believing that *they* know what is best for *you*. They are judgmental—judging people through their own experiences, from their particular point of view, recommending that the person with a problem fix it by doing what they would do, usually throwing in an "It's easy." On the plus side, egocentrics can pick themselves up by their bootstraps; on the negative side, they expect that everyone else can too.

As you might expect, egocentrics make lousy caretakers, their help too often limited to their way of seeing things. Lacking empathy, they see the problems of others as weakness, and difficulties in getting along as the other's fault. Egocentric parents, as prime producers of egocentric and neurotically dysfunctional children, are among society's biggest problems. They certainly are their children's biggest problem.

Any neurotic children out there? Take heart in the last sentence. Most likely it's your parents' fault. Although, just because it isn't your fault, doesn't mean that you're not the one stuck with patching yourself up.

Neurotics interacting with the world conversely find everything bad *their* fault, while minimizing their contribution to anything positive that happens. They are always coming up short in their own eyes. "I should have done this differently," "If only I had done that,"

"They probably won't like me," and "I'm sorry" are common laments of neurotics.

Low self-esteem, high levels of guilt, loneliness (even in company), and battles with depression are some characteristics of neurotic people.

Neurotics have their own problems with parenting. They tend to give too much in the parent/child relationship, are easily manipulated with guilt, and are generally poor role models for learning self-esteem. Neurotic parents have a similarly damaging propensity to rear egocentric and neurotic children of their own. Their children either find egocentric power in their abilities to manipulate the parent, or a lack of self-esteem through the parent's insecure modeling, or, and often, both.

Unfortunately, people at opposite ends of the egocentric-neurotic continuum often wind up partnered to one another. They are a tragic natural match. The egocentric deflects criticism and abuse, the neurotic absorbs it. Once accepted in a family unit, the dysfunctional hierarchy is established: Beginning with the egocentric, and in descending order, the neurotic, followed by the progeny. The best way out is to get fixed before you buy in. People with good self-esteem AND empathy are not cowed by the egocentric and can usually help the neurotic.

The good news for neurotics is that therapists can help them. Neurotics feel there is something wrong with them, so they are generally willing to try to fix it. And you can be fixed.

On the other hand, egocentrics don't think they have a problem—it's the world's fault—so they don't think they need help. The pain they generate is inflicted elsewhere, and since they don't feel it, they have trouble seeing the need to repair their "generator."

The egocentric-neurotic continuum does have a broad healthy center. This area is characterized by the balanced realization that I'm OK and we're all doing the best we can, and that people aren't better or worse than one another, just different. The healthy balancing of self-respect and respect for others makes a fairly good definition of sanity. Imagine, sane parents producing sane children. What a concept. Give it a try when your turn comes around.

Taking note of the many human contrasts can be very helpful. Getting caught in any few of them or in constant comparison in general is a waste. Through narrow comparison we may find one person beautiful, making another ugly; one's point of view right, another's therefore wrong. Isolating contrast, and that is the only way to draw contrast, ignores the wholer reality, creating a distortion without the recognition of a whole that is much more complex. Different musical notes in isolation can be more or less pleasing, but creatively combined, these notes make beautiful music. Life is most beautiful in harmony, not in petty isolation. Strive toward harmony. Be a part of the music.

Point of View (P.O.V.)

YOU are your point of view. From your brain, through your functioning sensory organs, from where you are at any given time, in any given place, all that you are, and the sum of your experiences help to shape your point of view. If you don't have a very accurate idea of where you are, what your vantage point is in this cosmic circus, your point of view ain't likely to be too accurate. For some in the "I-got-mine, don't-bother-me-with-this-shit, I'm-too-busy, head-stuck-firmly-up-my-ass" types this is not a problem. For the rest of us, knowing from whence we came and where we are is relevant.

Most agree that there are better P.O.V.s than others. Broad is generally and usually better than narrow. Having a sense or understanding of the realityscape, and some of the parameters of your P.O.V. within it, is important to increasing the accuracy of your perspective. It is not unlike making the course correction from magnetic north to north when plotting a nautical course, only in this case your P.O.V. is often the magnet requiring the correction. Just as we should be wary of the information a used-car salesman gives us about a car he is selling, we must be careful not to deceive ourselves into a rationalization of what is fair and what is best for us, or what is best for us right now and what is best for us in the long run. An example of the former might be, "If I am privileged, should I willingly give up some of that privilege to promote fairness?" An example of the latter: "Should I study now, or go to the party?" If you begin your thought process thinking you're not where you are, playing the fool, you're likely to stay a fool.

Dont'cha be no fool.

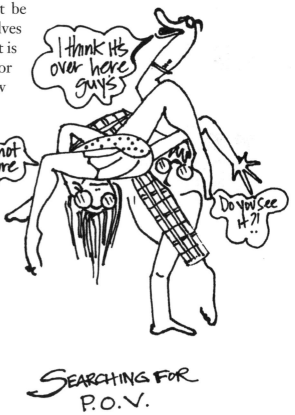

SEARCHING FOR P.O.V.

Heroes

There are essentially two kinds of heroes in this life.

The more commonly recognized hero is the person who dares to die; who risks his or her own life and personal safety to save or protect another. This is real heroism, but it is not the only kind.

The less popular form of heroism is to dare to live. People with this type of heroism daily live lives of integrity and contribution. They dare to stand or speak out against injustice even when perpetuating that injustice may benefit them. They daily present their best contribution to family and wider community, seldom needing more in return than the nourishment to continue. Taking only what they need, they always leave a surplus for those less fortunate or able.*

The measures of this type of heroism are more difficult to determine. We are all complicated mixes of strengths and weaknesses.

---

* In case any of you haven't noticed, I'm leaving out the sports hero. When the success of Michael Jordan's next jump shot is riding on something more important than the agony of de feet, I'll put the jocks back on the pedestal with real heroes.

Heroes who dare to live bring constant effort and honest appraisal to their affairs. They are open to ideas and information that might alter their point of view. Their goal is honest understanding. What they most want to know is what they may be most wrong about so that they can more accurately adjust their path and their thinking.

They also realize that we all walk in our own individual shoes. They try to understand and empathize with others. When the difficulty of understanding is too much, they strive, in their uncertainty, to trust the other person. Resisting the urge to judge others, refusing to allow themselves to be judg*mental*, they find that others, when trusted and respected, rarely abuse that trust. Through this simple act of trust, they are rewarded with cooperation, a profit that all may share.

Our society does a good job of valuing the positive contributions of people to this life, but is not very good at weighing contribution against personal deficit. It is in the balance sheet that the real measure of worth is found.

Let me give some examples:

We adore the player who hits the home run in the big game, but are not so critical if he neglects his family responsibilities.

We value corporate leaders who accomplish great profitability for shareholders by "downsizing," too often forgetting the uglier reality that this term has for so many affected families.

The "dare to live hero" isn't blinded by the bright lights, and refuses to use the backs of others as a ladder.

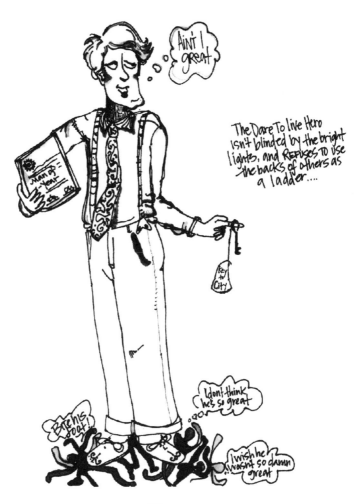

Masturbation & Morality

First let me say that I support masturbation, encourage it, advocate in its favor, am sympathetic to it, want it, need it, recommend it to the young, middle-aged and old, friends and foes alike, women and men, gays, bis, lesbians, heteros, transgenders, the able, the physically and mentally challenged, in fact, with rare exceptions due to critical physical problems, to everybody—and their dogs and cats and birds too. Just so you have an idea where I stand on this.

Some great sage of the 60's said, "If it feels good, do it." Though this may be a little over the top applied to everything that might feel good to everybody, it is perfectly accurate for masturbation. The better saying may be from the late mother of a dear friend. Grandmama Hirschman said, "There is no such thing as a bad orgasm."

The ONLY drawbacks to masturbation are of the psycho social variety: Negative and erroneous information instilled in you, by word and deed, by your parents, preachers and various and sundry other misguided moralists.

Masturbation has been alleged to cause blindness, acne, hair growth on the palms of your hands, sterility, fetal deformity, and dementia. Masturbation does none of these things, nor will it induce lightning to strike the spot of an unabetted tryst. What it will do is give you a fair amount of pleasure for the effort, and give a measure of peace to raging hormones. It can do many other beneficial things, but these are mostly gender specific, so I have divided the body of the essay into sections on women's and men's masturbation.

Comparing male and female sexuality is a fool's errand. We are different in fundamental ways and in innumerable other significant ways. This contrast is just another prime example of the futility of attempts at broad learning through narrow comparison. I have divided gender specific information on masturbation into two separate parts quite simply because we are so different. That doesn't mean there's no connection. There is a wonderful connection.

Women

There are many reasons why a woman's sexual satisfaction has been ignored by Western Civilization, but let's start with the guys who wrote the Bible. Old Testament, New Testament, doesn't matter, it's all a testament to how a dominant special interest group—

men—ignored the needs and best interests of a (supposedly) lesser group—women—for THOUSANDS OF YEARS!!!

The Bible isn't the only place this male dominant philosophy was played out. The Koran, the Islamic holy book, is quite similar in its sexual chauvinism. I'm not sure, but my guess is that these convergent points of view were more the result of sexually unenlightened guys writing the different texts than the divine word of a sexually unenlightened God dude.

Anyway, this little arrangement was institutionalized in Western (and Middle Eastern) civilization. It says in the Bible and the Koran and still in most legal statutes everywhere that missionary position copulation for the purposes of procreation is the only "approved" type of sex. Everything else, everything that might require extra effort in a man, or provide satisfaction for a women, was immoral, illegal, *unnatural*, and Bad!

Traditional Judeo-Christian teachings about sexuality originated and have been perpetuated in a paternalistically hierarchical culture where the interests of women have been ignored. To mix a couple of metaphors, that shit no longer floats, and Jeanie ain't goin back in the bottle. ANY (old or new) rational theology or philosophy regarding what is best for society must be a joint effort of masculine and feminine thought. Any teaching on what is in the best interests of women sexually must be firmly controlled by women, certainly not by what a bunch of long-dead men from a patriarchal past proclaimed for them.

At the beginning of the Industrial Age and with the flourishing of science, liberated eggheads finally began to scientifically prove why everything that happens happens. Naturally, mostly scientific *men* began to study sexuality. In denial about their personal experience, they once again proved what they were already wrong about: during the mid-19th century, doctors, upon observing institutionalized female mental patients masturbating, concluded that this was the probable root of their dementia. The other possible observable conclusion, that these poor women were just making the best of a bad situation, for some reason never occurred to them.

A few decades later Sigmund Freud got involved. Siggy was one helluva dude, for a dude. He figured out more stuff about the mind than all the shrinks before him put together. But like any smart guy, he occasionally got a little too far ahead of himself, and, like the good doctors over at the insane asylum and most social scientists to this day, he often didn't take into account the personal baggage, his own prejudices and predilections, that he brought to his analyses.

Freud deduced that a young girl's sexual feelings were strongest in the clitoris, but that as she matured they moved to her vagina. Whoops, old Siggy let a little wishful thinking slip in there. Of course if you're a guy, you can see why a woman's erogenous zone should be in her vagina, that's where we're equipped to do our best work. Too bad it ain't so.

Today, a male-dominant sexual confusion is still the cultural mainstay for our attitudes on sex as we vaingloriously march into the 21st century.

As Thea Lowry, the wonderfully insightful sex therapist instructs, "Although sex is perfectly natural, it is not always naturally perfect."

Man puts his penis in a woman's vagina. It feels great (for a man), and every now and then she gets pregnant and has a baby. About half the time it's a boy. That's where the saying "Oh Boy" comes from. Somehow "Oh Girl" hasn't caught on yet. No matter that a woman's prime area of sexual arousal is her clitoris, a beensy little organ that gets precious little attention from penile pistoning of the vagina. So the traditional love act is not necessarily very stimulating to women. There is good reason for this relevant to survival of the species. If a women more easily reached orgasm through penile vaginal insertion, men might not reach orgasm before the women pushed them off and contentedly went to sleep (sound familiar here?). There would be no male ejaculation, no sperm attack on the fallopian tubes, no accidents of pregnancy, and possibly no continued accident of humanity.

Looking at all this, it is easy to see—if not easy to deal with the anger—how women's sexual satisfaction has been mostly MIA for several thousand years now. So what's a modern woman to do? Simple answer: take matters into her own hands. Don't hesitate, masturbate.

The Declaration of Independence says that all people have the right to life, liberty and the pursuit of happiness. So, if you consider yourself a member in good standing of this group—all people—you have the right to the pursuit of happiness. Since masturbation is the primary way women first experience orgasm, and since few things are as pleasing to a woman as an orgasm, the Declaration of Independence CALLS UPON YOU TO MASTURBATE.

The reason that masturbation is so important for women is that your clitoris and your orgasm aren't so easy to find, especially with our cultural aversion to them.

Women come in all varieties (say Hallelujah!). Their sexuality is as varied as the differences of how they look, feel and think, but if you have a clitoris, and the time, with extremely rare exceptions, all women can become orgasmic.

Learning about masturbation if you have never tried it, or have been unsuccessful trying it (for any of many wonderfully under-standable reasons) is easy. I am certainly not the best person to give this advice, but there are plenty of women who are. Talk to other women. The word is definitely getting out. Or read some of the many books now in print. A group situation is also a great way for pre-orgasmic women to share their fears and insights and to support one another. College campuses are an extremely conducive place for these group gatherings. It is the first time young women are away from home, with an opportunity to think and act freely. I am frankly surprised that there are not more opportunities on campus for women to explore their sexuality in this way.

For those whose enjoyment, or even the contemplation of mas-turbation and sexual pleasure, is blocked by psychic scarring, please, *read the literature and seek help*. All of the scholarly work on sexuali-ty agrees on the efficacy (that's a good thing) of masturbation in human sexuality. It is morally good, spiritually good, emotionally good, physically good, civically good, and naturally good.

OK, let's get to a few last details before we conclude again with the main theme of this essay: that masturbation and sexual satisfaction are good, good, good.

Stereotype-shattering anthropologist Margaret Mead long ago reported that in cultures where female orgasm is considered important, the essential techniques which will lead to orgasm will be part of the teachings of that culture. If female orgasm is not considered important, there will be little emphasis on teaching about it.

When we realized 500 years ago that the world wasn't flat, we began to make adjustments. What say we keep spreading the word about female sexuality. Men were better off when they stopped worrying about falling off the end of the earth; we can adjust to this too. Since it may take another 500 years, we better get started, but first men, let's see who else besides me wants to be a jerk off.

Men

I first had sex when I was about 12 or 13 in a cubbyhole in the basement of my friend Gerry's house. We knew it was supposed to be wrong. Our parents, teachers and preachers said so. Ah, the shame of it, or should I say, ahhhhhHHHHHHHHHHhhh, the shame of it! I had sex several more times before a partner finally joined me about five years later, but sadly I missed out on much more sexual release because of fears of lightning, hairy palms, or the social pathology that accompanied the moniker "jerk off." "Not me babe. I may have the bluest balls in the county—sometimes it felt like the whole universe—but I am no jerk off." Well, it turns out that it does take one to know one. I was a jerk off (= a fool) for not jerking myself off! Good thing I wasn't hung up about nose picking, I'd have really gone crazy!

Masturbation does two things for a guy. It relieves sexual tension—no small matter for you younger guys, and it can help you learn how to control your ejaculation when you do get lucky—no small matter for any guy. In fact, masturbating to learn how to become a better lover is a win/win/win situation, at the least:

The first win is it's FUN and FEELS GOOD!

Second win is that you get to practice ejaculation control and make mistakes without embarrassing yourself or your partner. "Oops, oh well, have to take a nap and try again later."

Third win: If you've vented your raging hormones sufficiently, you won't seem like such a Horn Dog to a girl you like.

I don't have much more to say. For guys and masturbation there isn't that much to say. Throw in a partner though and it's a whole new ball game, if you know what I mean. In this brave new world you can't just masturbate into your woman and get away with it. Women, now finally free of the inferiority crap this patriarchal culture has been shoveling since Christ knows when, don't need us any more than we need them. Maybe less. The myths of male superiority and female inferiority are DEAD. This is a good thing, even if it means that men will have to change, will have to learn how to be full partners, will have to realize that their greatest and lasting pleasure lies in giving pleasure.

Men are not intimidated by female sexuality or sexually assertive partners if they have learned how to be successful partners. So guys, if you haven't read carefully, go back and read about women and masturbation and also "Love and Sex." The real stud muffins in this world don't kid themselves because they realize that they can't kid their partners. Learn how to be a good partner and the world will be a happier place, and you'll be happier in it.

Stuff

WESTERN
MEDITATION

When I was 18 years old, I realized what an idiot I had been at 17, and how much more together I was at 18.

When I was 19, I had a similar revelation.

Funny, but at 20 the genius of 19 in retrospect became a fool, replaced by a new improved genius, and a real man.

Now, nearing 50 I am really grown up—I think.

The Clone

Everybody's got their own version of fate's fickle finger; of how our actions are intermeshed with the known and unknown forces of existence.

In India, most people believe that there is a cosmic accounting ledger that keeps track of the good and bad things we do in life. Like Santa, when we were kids, it credits or debits each person for all the naughty or nice things he or she does. Your balance sheet is known as your karma.

In Ireland, a land of warm beer and damp, foggy weather, a more pessimistic, though pragmatic, attitude prevails. Murphy's Law instructs us to expect the worst, and we won't be disappointed.

Hollywood has always produced its own version of this cosmic force. The Good Guys have it and the Bad Guys don't. "The Force" in "Star Wars" is an elaborate take-off on this simplistic idea.

Humans everywhere feebly and futilely attempt to grasp and understand the ungraspable and unknowable. In the summer of 1970, Phroggie, Mescaline Mouse, Krinkle, Grit, Roger Ramjet,

Weird George, and the other denizens of Sea View Avenue joined the fray with a version of their own called The Clone.

No one recalls how it came to be called "The Clone." No one recalls too much from those days. Someone thought it might have had to do with cloning luck, and therefore, staying lucky, though no one else thought it had anything at all to do with cloning anything. When I asked Uncle Al—a revered member of the Sea View Avenue days—about it, he observed, "Why did they call golf 'golf?'" His explanation, that it was because the word "shit" was already taken, may say more about him than the origin of the clone.

No one can understand the clone completely, or should try to— it's all in that dancing too close to the flame thing—but we do know a few things about it. The clone flows through some combination of luck, karma, intuition, humility, and "the right timing of useful deeds."

Sometimes, just sitting around, you can get some good clone; like if somebody smashes into your car in the same spot where you smashed it up the week before. In this way the clone is like luck. Having your car hit, usually a bad thing, but hit where you just messed it up, that's pure clone, or pure luck.

The clone likes folks better when they're young. This is a

karmic thing. Young people haven't had as much time to do bad stuff. In fact, babies have the best clone (in all things except who their parents are, even the clone can't do anything about that). When you're young sometimes it's fun to fuck around with the clone. You know, drive too fast, take some chances. Usually the clone doesn't mind, as long as you don't get too nasty, or too selfish, or *too unlucky*.

Intuition is a big part of the clone. The clone knows when you're trying too hard, or are sucking up to it, and when it's just you being good folks. It is no fan of do-gooders—folks just trying to get to heaven. Random acts of kindness are one thing. Random acts of kindness, done with the idea that this'll get you some good clone, can be very bad clone.

The clone involves a lot of luck, but you can increase the odds of getting and keeping it by doing the right thing. There's a saying, "Where preparation meets opportunity lies fortune," which means you can play a part in making your own luck. In concert, Janis Joplin, in her lead-in to the song "Try a Little Bit Harder," used to tell the story about how a woman who lived downstairs from her always had more boyfriends. Janis couldn't figure it out until she came home about seven or eight one morning, and passed the woman, who was headed out onto the street. That babe was getting out on the street four or five hours ahead of Janis. She was giving herself more time to get lucky.

This is the coolest part of the clone. Just simple stuff, doing the right thing at the right time, time and again, begins over time to become magical. If you're working hard, doing the right thing, if you understand and practice **prevention,** are attentive and caring with others and other things, when you need something to happen for you, **way opens.** Your good clone rewards you. Just don't count on it. Like the rest of the *fates,* de clone don't like no arrogance.

You can keep the clone by doing the right thing, but it's not necessarily your idea of the right thing, it's the clone's. So you have to keep checking to see if your idea of the right thing is really the right thing.

Good clone can be a remedy to the modern perversions Mark Twain so eloquently wrote about over a century ago. People with the clone allow "soft romance" and simple "contentment" to ward off "vulgar ambitions" and "vicious appetites." They sleep better too.

You can have the clone your whole life, if you work at it daily, best you can.

Bad clone is easier to get, just start screwing up, getting greedy, or taking shortcuts with your partners.

Sometimes good folks, doing the right thing, get some bad clone. Sometimes you just have to ride it out. Other times you have to reach way down to see if the bad clone seed is deep inside you.

I'd wish all of you good clone, but you all know it'd just be a jive gesture, something like "Have a nice day."

The Spirit of Life

All human life has a common spirit, a common consciousness, a common origin. Everyone starts life with this purity of consciousness. Each life stems from this common wellspring to become its own individual existence based on the myriad factors that shape each of us.

Whatever a person does, at any moment in life, is likely how the *origin* of your consciousness would react in dem same shoes. And whatever you do—great, grandiose or gross, is probably what any other human consciousness would accomplish/do having traveled to the same point in your skin.

Realizing that what any other person is doing at any given time is likely what the origin of your consciousness would be doing if dealt the same hand is basic to human understanding, tolerance and respect.

Human differences all stem from this common origin. Based on genetics, nutrition, nurturing, and no little bit of experiential fortune, we are shaped. The story of the Prince and the Pauper attempts to explain this metaphorically, as do many other similar folk histories. This is one of the few metaphysical markers that stands up to all the proofs we can apply. As a purely spiritual matter, NO ONE IS BETTER OR WORSE THAN ANYONE ELSE!

Personal Responsibility

Just because where you are is most likely where any other consciousness would be in this life of yours, doesn't mean that you have no control over your future.

And, just as it may not be your fault how you got to be this person that you are, you are now the one in charge.

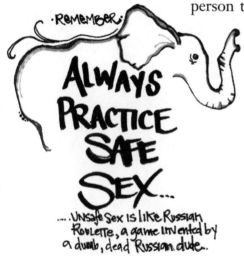

Whatever you do for or to yourself, or someone else, is *your* responsibility.

It is now *your* job to find out who you are, what is right with you, and what may be broken, or torn, or disoriented. But that doesn't mean you have to do it alone. Often you can't do it alone.

We need each other.

Ask for help.

The Disinformation Age

Back when I was coming of age—way, way back—in the 60s, there was a faith similar to today's in the media's ability to lead us toward our higher ideals. Today we see TV ads of diverse, beautiful, smiling faces from around the world sharing the internet. In the psychedelic 60s, a fellow named Marshall McLuhan was considered a visionary voice promising that new media advances would lead us toward a new global harmony. Then, much like today, people wanted to believe that new technology would solve our human problems.

Media advances can and do help reduce parochialism, help people to understand that there is a great deal more to life than their tiny corner of it. But media advances have an off-setting downside. In creating mind-boggling profitability, they have changed any semblance of a noble fourth estate into a ruthless bottom-line megaindustry. The supposed people's watchdog of government and other rich and powerful special interests is now a full-fledged member of these groups. Today our media is little more than the PR branch of the corporate-state that is our reality. Its chief products are a society-numbing crass commercialism, it's-not-our-fault news, and a consumer homogenization that has been called the Los Angelization of America, or, and perhaps more appropriately, the malling of the world.

Let's take a short look back at how we got here, and where we are, relevant to you.

I remember the first time I heard about Marshal McLuhan's most famous work, *The Medium Is the Message*. I very astutely pondered, "What the hell is that?" and "Marshall of What?"

Anyway, McLuhan became fabulously famous for a single erudite thought. In the blooming information age—back in the 60s it was flowers, today we're talking algae with a bullet—the volume of the media would dwarf in significance any particular message or messages it would convey.

Of course, like any academic worth his salt, he immediately and feverishly wrote a series of books that erroneously applied this principle to all of history, and made even more foolish predictions about the future.

Historically, he postulated that the primary method of mass communication in any era was the most important aspect in shaping the character of that era. (See his seminal work: *Were the Indians Just Blowing Smoke?*)

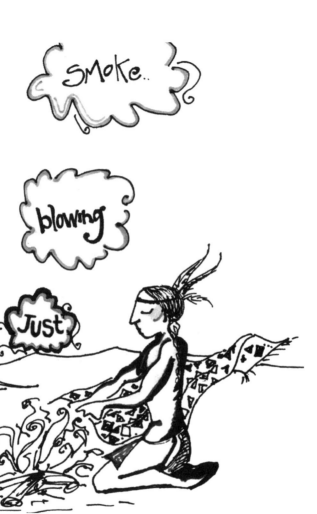

His erroneous extrapolations about the future were that these newly interconnected and incredibly rapid electronic media would lead to an end of individualism and nationalism, and usher in a melding of international communities and utopian cooperation. Unfortunately for the good professor, he was an academic marshall, never needing to ride reality's range. What actually happened was very close to what he thought, but as we soon learn, the devil is in the details.

Those who had control over the media would have power over those who had insights to relevant truths in the emerging dis-Information Age. It is becoming ever less important how valid what you say is, and ever more important to how many people and how many times you can afford to say it.

McLuhan missed such details as the free market's interest in the profitability of the emerging media industry, entrenched power's interests, and stuff like that. In this bottom-line world, newspapers, news magazines and TV news rooms are less controlled by journalists than by corporate managers and marketers.

Newspapers and magazines that sacrifice the whims and prejudices of their core readerships for an unvarnished truth face swiftly declining subscriptions. TV newscasts that don't pander to the broadest demographic segments of their audiences face falling ratings and revenues.

Half-truth, hyperbole, pandering, self-aggrandizement, and bald-faced lying have become an accepted part of the fabric of our lives. Everybody with something to sell has learned "spin." And everybody has something to sell: politicians (why do they always come up?), religions (they can't all be right), institutes of higher education (We're perfect for you. Pick us), boys (I love you), girls (of course these are real), the army, navy, air force and marines (ever been in one of them?), EVERYFUCKINGBODY lies. It's no longer caveat emptor—let the buyer beware—it's caveat everybody and everything.

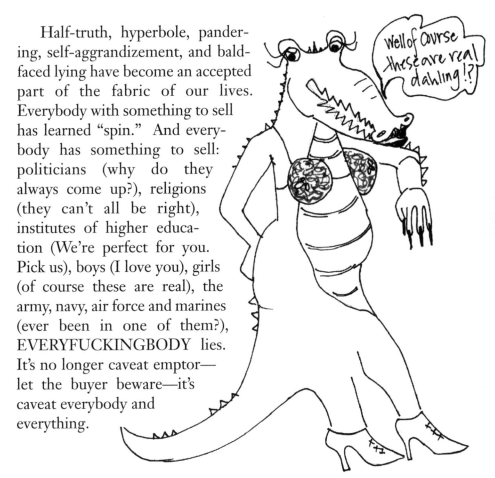

99

The better you do it, the better you do. You know the financier's credo: "The key to success in life is sincerity. Once you learn to fake that, the rest is easy."

So what can you do? It's a corrupt world out there. Should you just get wasted, jam your head firmly in the sand, sell out yourself, become a communist, join the Sisyphus Society, end the misery and pull the plug?

Wait! It's not that bad. Just send $14.95 to me at...just kidding. What you have to do is develop a finely honed shit detector. It's not that hard to do, and there are some handy hints to help you along the way, but it takes time (ugh), patience (double ugh), and effort (spoken like the true old fart that I am).

It's a back-to-basics, back-to-nature kind of a thing. And there is not much hierarchy to the rules of shit detection. Personal integrity through serious introspection, however, is the best foundation.

When I was about thirteen, my dad took me on a fishing trip. On that trip at one point he told me that I was the last arbiter of the truth. Not him, or mom, or any other authority figure. He said that all individuals had a right to find their own truths, and that although they had no monopoly on them, neither did anybody else.

Whatever else my old man told me, he was right-on about this. The first big step is being honest with yourself. Once you've come clean with yourself—no small order for all you living-large-inside-the-bubble types—shit detection is a fairly simple process. Weigh what is said versus the possible motives of the person who is saying it.

Next, don't give up on the possibility of trusting others; just be careful. Hey, this whole thing didn't just happen. People have been getting suckered ever since Ug clubbed his pal Mug to steal Jugs. Make friends slowly. Don't risk more than you can lose. If it sounds too good to be true, IT IS! Pay your way: There is No free lunch. And, most of all, be honest with yourself. Lao Tzu knew it best when he said, "How do I know this integrity? Because it could all begin in me."

If that doesn't work for you, flash 'em your pearliest whites and lie like a rug. What the hell, everybody else does.

The Myopia of Upward Mobility

The sanest person realizes that nobody has an absolute right to shit in this cruel world. If not caught in a war, starving, physically or mentally crippled, sick, in jail, or freezing their ass off, they're thanking Christ for their good fortune in the scheme of things.

We live in such a bountiful society. Things are so good that we lose the awareness of how far down it can go from here, how much farther down it is for most in the human condition. Instead, most of us have this character flaw that only lets us see how much better things should be.

Consider this:

Eight percent of the world's families own a car.

Affluent American children spend more in pocket money per year ($750) than a quarter of the world's poorest families earn in the same time.

Since 1940 Americans have used up as much of the earth's mineral resources as everyone before them combined.

What is this flaw in the human psyche that only allows so many to see how much better things could be, that allows us to forget how much worse things can get, how much more fortunate we are than so many others, or how much happier we could be if we realized our good fortune?

This *strain* of thought continues, making it much easier for us to see what's wrong with the other person, instead of ourselves. It allows us to accept unfair advantage, if we are the recipients, rather than to stand for fairness, even at our own expense.

This egocentricity can make anyone think they are better than anyone else. The same flaw is found in belief in the superiority of one religion over another, one race or ethnicity over another, and one gender over another.

Doing well, at bottom, has more to do with your birthright and good fortune than anything else. Realizing this, all of the great mystics taught that the highest of people were also the humblest. There, but for the twist of fate, go I.

The commonality of the human experience is our Rosetta Stone, not our false attempts at elitist distinction.

Homosexuality

One man puts his penis into another man's anus. People who don't do this usually find it repugnant to even think about.

Women who are romantically and sexually attracted to other women often satisfy each other through oral stimulation of the clitoris. Many people are offended by the thought of this also.

When I go to the mall, and observe the Sea of Humanity in all its glory, were I to imagine many of the heterosexual couples I encounter engaged in their idea of sex, it might repulse the shit out of me too. I do not propose harm be done to these people. Just that they, like everyone else, do it in private. If not, I will, whenever possible, be happy to look the other way.

Homosexuality is threatening to so many people, not because it is a real danger to them, but because it exposes a matrix of ignorance, revulsion and hypocrisy that has been culturally imbued in them, that people don't want to, or usually have to, deal with. And because they fear, rightly or wrongly, that they could somehow have an affinity for this seemingly repulsive behavior.

Sexually Transmitted Dis-Ease

Homosexuality is not a pathology (a mental or physical illness), it is—get ready for this one—just DIFFERENT! It is our society that is dis-eased by homosexuality, not homosexuality that is a disease.

Today, these are quite easy statements to make. The evidence is overwhelming and clear, but it hasn't always been so. About twenty years ago the psychiatric and psychological communities removed homosexuality from the lists of pathological disorders, recognizing it as alternative, as opposed to deviant, sexual behavior. For most of the twentieth century our mental health professionals erroneously defined homosexuality as a psychological disorder. Combined with the prejudicial dogma heaped on by our mainline religions, homosexuality became an easy whipping boy for society; a society that had come to be predicated on the comforts of hierarchy. In America, most folks stayed happy because most of us had people below us to kick around and be superior to. Folks who wound up at the end of this line either "brought it on themselves"—i.e. "perverted homosexuals," or were portrayed as simply inferior—women, minorities and the disabled.

Make no mistake about who the primary victims of this hierarchical abuse have been, but remember that we are all victimized by cultural xenophobia that turns human differences into devaluing pathologies, debilities, sins and crimes. Homophobic people have also been unfairly and unfortunately conditioned to this mind-set.

Improving the health of society does not entail making people who are homosexual heterosexual, or making everyone who is not white act in the custom of the white minority (whites are a small minority of the *earth's* people); or making left-handed people right-handed—though these have all been tried by people claiming the high moral and intellectual ground. ***Society will become healthier as we learn to accept the realities of human difference.*** Society will progress when we realize that human difference is not a better or worse proposition, just fucking different, or in this case, just different fucking.

Do Gooders

There is a general rule of thumb that folks who act 'holier than thou' are more likely to be caught in some nefarious deed. There's good reason that clergy, and other extollers of pure virtue, regularly come undone. Trying to be too good—superhumanly good—is extremely stressful. It robs people of the naturalness of being themselves, replacing it with artificial and unnatural expectations. Many people crack under the strain of having to be too good.

The logic of these "do gooders" is for others to do the same: for people to act just like them, or more accurately, the way they say we should be, for homosexuals to act heterosexual, for non-whites to act with Euro sensibilities.

As a groovy fairly happy heterosexual with a fine and reciprocating love partner, imagine how you would feel having to stay away from that partner, and to have to take on a same-sex lover, or be ostracized by your society. Homosexuals are *naturally* as repulsed by heterosexuality as the good hetero burghers are of gay/lesbian sex.

Ironically for gays and lesbians, there's a group for them to kick around too: bisexuals. Just as people in many cultures ostracize mixed ethnicity children, bisexuals are often shunned by the homosexual community. Homosexuals don't believe that these folks are really bi, assuming that they must be lesbians or gays in denial, or confusion. So everybody's sexually scared of, or hostile toward, someone else for no good reason. There are bad reasons though, most having to do with acculturations that inculcate us with suspicion toward human difference, ignorance and fear about sexuality, and a paranoia about strangers. Most of us today are uneasy in the presence of strangers. The Unitarian Universalist Minister Roy Phillips has written,

> We often feel uncomfortable with strangers—they are unknowns, strangers are formless personalities to us. We don't know what to expect so we make things up. The stranger is a Rorschach inkblot upon whom we project what is deeper down within us.

One of the primary things 'deep down within us' in this culture is an ignorance, confusion and fear about sexuality, so the stranger with a different sexuality opens a caldron of fears *within* us. Since society has sanctioned this fear of the stranger and fear of sexuality with nefarious platitudes like "family values" and "the American Way," and the media often sensationalize human anomaly, it becomes easier to scapegoat other people for their differences than to take the responsibility for repairing that which is deep within us. Blaming "others" for our own shortcomings has a long (sad) human history.

The Religious Wrong

The more fundamentalist Christians and Jews have had a particularly hard time trying to unlearn their homophobias. They have had the additional burden of exaggerated scriptural interpretation of the Bible's archaic passages condemning homosexuality. Though the Old Testament scriptures clearly reject homosexuality, there are many more passages that condone slavery, approve of racial segregation and polygamy, allow women to be men's property, and call for the death of interest-charging money lenders. Yet, the ban against homosexuality is the only one of these still held as sacrosanct. It is the only one that has not been rejected as an obsolete cultural overlay of that ancient time and place. So the Bible, a book that even amateur theologians know can be interpreted to conform to almost any madness—Nazi Germany was a Christian nation—has been used as a homophobic tool against its own higher teachings.

Jesus, who spoke regularly of the impossibility of the rich attaining salvation, had nothing to say about homosexuality. No wonder rich Christians are so homophobic. They're trying to keep the real Christian heat off their own asses. And finally, *Jesus' primary message was one of overcoming all hate and prejudice with an ever-expanding, all inclusive, universal love.* There is no asterisk that says except homosexuals, or except anyone else, for that matter.

Hetero Mythology

"Well, what about the fact that it's unnatural to be homosexual?" some might be asking.

It is NOT unnatural. Homosexuality, in the sense of same sex sexual attraction, has always been present in humans. Its presence has been recorded since the beginning of written language 5000 years ago in (the original) Babylon. It was present in all of the other "cradle" civilizations of the world: Egyptian, Indian, Chinese, and Mayan.

It has been observed in the animal world in domestic animals (bulls, cows, stallions, donkeys, cats, rams, goats, and pigs), and in the wild in antelope, elephants, hyenas, chimpanzees, monkeys, apes, rabbits, lions, porcupines, hamsters, mice and porpoises. Bisexuality and hermaphrodites are necessities that underpin evolution in lower phylum animals and the entire vegetative and sub-vegetative world. One thing that homosexuality is NOT is unnatural.

"Well, aren't homosexuals more likely to molest my children?"

No. The main statistical correlations to predatory child sexual abuse are maleness and having been a victim of abuse as a child. Ninety percent of child sexual abuse is committed by heterosexual men, and most of that upon those in their care. Sexual deviance is part of the vicious cycle of child abuse: vulnerable children, cruelly treated, later repeat that pathology in adulthood, on other unfortunate children.

"Won't homosexuals turn children into homosexuals?"

This more interesting question leads back to broader cultural, rather than any inherent homosexual, perversion.

First and primarily, sexual orientation is determined by romantic attraction. I don't know about you, but my romantic attraction has always been a very innate thing. I know from painful experience that the most powerful and trusted people in my life have had no luck whatsoever in dissuading me from my, often poor, romantic choices.

This does not imply, however, that a person's sexuality is entirely immutable, or immune to environmental forces. B. F. Skinner and his pals showed how behavior modification can be powerfully accomplished. Alcohol and other drugs create monumental changes in human behavior. Why are most of the people in Christian culture Christian, while most in Muslim culture are Muslim, if not for the power of cultural conditioning? Just as there are many homosexuals culturally pressed into an unhappy heterosexuality, heterosexuals can be driven into an unhappy homosexuality. Children from abusive families can have a wide range of outcomes to their experiences. A normally heterosexual young boy can be alienated from women by an abusive and domineering mother. Many young women find male sexual contact traumatic because their fathers raped them. These children could well be more susceptible to an unnatural homosexuality.

Charges of sodomizing boys, and of turning young girls into lesbians, have been used as principle moral weapons against homosexuals. There are severe problems with this type of hysteria. It is mostly the societal magnification of the prejudicial label "homosexual predators," as opposed to the more germane "sexual predators." Gays and lesbians are no more likely to be deviant than anyone else. More important for society is the continued difficulty in protecting children's welfare without unduly infringing upon legitimate parental rights, for it is in the home where the overwhelming amount of perversion and abuse is perpetuated. Unloving, cruel, and dysfunctional environments propel the downward spiral toward sexual deviance. None of this has to do with a person's innate sexual orientation, homo or hetero.

"AIDS is God's revenge against homosexuality."

Does that mean that God's chosen ones are lesbians, who have the lowest risk of contracting AIDS (or any sexually transmitted disease)? Or perhaps it means, correspondingly, that syphilis, gonorrhea, the crabs and herpes are God's revenge against heterosexuals. This would make God into some sort of sexual sociopath, with lesbians as His chosen ones, wouldn't it?

Many worry that if society sanctioned homosexuality and bisexuality that there would be an increase in the two. I believe this is true. Societal repression does keep people from enjoying their nonconforming romantic and sexual desires. There would probably be some increase in the homosexual population, though it is plain that humanity is preponderantly heterosexual. Acceptance would also lead to a decrease in teen suicide, a large portion of which is caused by young homosexuals caught in brutally homophobic environments. It would eliminate the terrible unhappiness and dysfunction that homophobic people must put themselves and their families through when they realize that a loved one is gay. And it would allow all of us to be more accepting of all difference, an ever-growing necessity in our ever-shrinking world.

So you tell me, is it wrong to be homosexual, or is it wrong to think it's wrong? Better yet, tell yourself, and then have the courage to tell the world.

A Velox Overlay of the Big Picture

Back in the pre-digital Dark Ages of printing, about 15 years ago, making a color photograph for a magazine or book required combining four different colored sheets of clear Velox plastic, overlayed on one another. Each colored transparency had a negative of the picture etched onto it: red, yellow, blue and green. Individually each sheet was just shades of its own color, and, like any film negative, somewhat difficult to distinguish, but when all four sheets were laid on top of one another over a white background, a clear color picture burst into view. It is in the combining of the four sheets that the one clear picture emerges.

Gaining understanding of individuals, or of any complex social system, is often best achieved by overlaying different dynamics on top of one other, like so many sheets of Velox are overlaid to make a color photo.

There is a type of Japanese dramatic play called a Roshimon that illustrates a similar point. In this type of play, the same drama is acted out over and over from the different points of view of each witness to the action. Any one section of the play gives a single, and somewhat distorted, point of view, but when all parts of the play are seen, and the audience has an opportunity to know each character and to see each one's point of view, a much clearer picture of what really transpired is revealed.

These are extremely valuable tools for understanding some of the complex parts of our complex world. Let's take a look at an application of the Velox overlay method and see how this works.

The example I have chosen is an individual's psychological profile. Please don't take my scientific characterizations too seriously though; I am to the study of psychology as a dead squirrel is to taxidermy.

To gain a broad understanding of an individual's psychological profile, you could begin with a Freudian analysis, overlay a Myers-Briggs personality assessment, determine the person's position on an egotistical/neurotic continuum, then landscape it with a little broad-brush physiology and anthropology.

Freud instructed us on the fundamental importance of life's first years, for example, how much the primary (Oedipal) relationships—mother and father to son and daughter—can dominate our sexuality and sense of well being throughout life.

The Myers-Briggs personality assessment attempts to describe the post-adolescent shake-out of predilections that will define us along four basic scales: introvert-extrovert, thinker-feeler, sensate-intuitive, and judging-perceiving.

The egotistical-neurotic continuum (previously described on pp. 65-69) determines much of who does what to who, and to what degree individuals are affected by their relationships with others.

Any of the three grids, accurately drawn, can give great insight into a person's psychological profile, but overlaid on one another, they flesh out the picture, enhancing and reinforcing the other individual parts.

The roles of physiology (your bio-chemistry and genealogy) would fill still more voids in the picture, and adding the story of a person's acculturation would make the picture damn near breathe.

There are many other important and valid psychological parameters that could be added to the "overlay," or perhaps substituted for some of these individual parts. What is significant is the need for multiple layers of information along different continuums for broad accurate mappings, and as proofs against the other findings relevant to the whole (in this case) person.

More practically, say your partner, for no good reason, acts as if he or she doesn't like you, when you seem to have done nothing wrong. If you are neurotic, any clues as to other reasons for this behavior will be quickly discarded in favor of the fact that your partner has finally realized what a loser you are. The problem could be bad Oedipal blood: your partner may just be projecting on to you some old rub with the same-sexed parent. Or it could be that his or her (Myers-Briggs) "feeler" is annoyed with your "thinker." Or, physiologically, maybe he or she is just feeling like shit that day. If you are open to many different possibilities you are more likely to discover the real problem.

The Roshimon and the colored plastic sheets thing are good examples of how to simply but effectively look at, and come to understand, complexity. Looking at one sheet of Velox, or one part of a Roshimon is incomplete, and simplistic. You don't have to be a genius to figure out lots of complicated things. You just have to know how to simply (rather than simplistically) try.

Politics

Remember all that stuff your parents and teachers taught you about our wonderful system of government? Mostly a bunch of crap. You know what the media tells you? About 90% crap. What politicians tell you about themselves? Pure crap.

Do you know why most Americans usually choose not to vote? Because they're smarter than the rest. They know the system is rigged, and their vote ain't worth a spit in the ocean.

Power and money have more to do with winning elections than individuals' votes. Been that way, more or less, since day one in this here U S of A. Let's take a few minutes to review American politics relative to the importance of your vote since when old George first said "I Do."

The Founding Buds

The Founding Fathers (note the absence of the mothers) did not establish a democracy, or even a republic, although that's what they called it. In reality, the great reform of America was from colonial rule by a monarchy to a liberal oligarchy where only some white men, usually landed and minimally of some means, could vote. They wrote and established a constitution that said something much different, but that was meant as a guideline for *future* reform after these old boys were gone.

You don't read much in the history books about how George Washington, Sam Adams (that's where that whiny dude got the name for his beer), Alexander Hamilton, or Tom Jefferson made decisions based on the will of the people. They were mostly influenced by each other. Al Hamilton expressed these feelings clearest when he wrote, "The voice of the people has been said to be the voice of God, and however generally this maxim has been quoted and believed, it is not true in fact. The people...seldom judge or determine right." Reading this it is not difficult to see why the first five American presidents were elected with something less than 1% of the white voting age male population. Not exactly what you'd call the Cradle of Democracy, unless of course, you were robbing that cradle.

Interestingly, the founding buds were not all that different in their view of how republican democracy would eventually flow from their enlightened oligarchy than Karl Marx was in expecting that an enlightened communist leadership would eventually "wither away."

The problem all of these eggheads overlooked was that people are very reluctant to give up their good thing. It's like trying to take a ball away from a kid when he knows everyone else wants it.

The biggest toughest smartest kid usually gets hold of the ball and keeps it till the next bigger badder kid comes along. Now that's political philosophy!

So, everybody meant well, but from George right through to today, nobody wants to share the ball, and they all basically use the same rationale: I'm smarter, so you should trust me. The proof is "I won," and now I've got the ball. The elitism of the winner is one of the prime factors that constantly queers our deal.

Everybody tells us George Washington really wanted to do the right thing by democracy, but he had start-up problems, so he had to put the good stuff on the back burner. Sam Adams we know was too busy making beer. When Tom Jefferson became president, he thought slavery was wrong but he couldn't get rid of it, he'd 'uv had about five hundred paternity suits filed against him by newly enfranchised citizens. James Madison was a liberal guy, but when he got a hold of the ball, suddenly sharing didn't seem so important.

Expanding the right to vote has been a grudgingly slow process ever since. Early on the federal government ceded to the individual states the power to determine eligibility to vote. The common hook was you had to be a white guy sitting on the same piece of rock for some time. In some states if you paid enough taxes (but only rented a condo) you could participate in our free and open democracy, in other places you had to belong to the right church too.

God Bless America
(As Soon as We Kill the Natives)

Andrew Jackson was the first guy to do any real damage to this cozy little rich guys' deal. As our first great populist, he realized, after getting trimmed by John Quincy Adams in 1824, the value of getting out the eligible vote. In 1828 he got out the vote in a big way, more than tripling the turnout to well over one million voters. (While lots of white men may have loved good ole Andy, he killed, displaced, and cheated way too many Native Americans to have much of a following with them, and the 150 or so slaves he owned at the time of his death probably weren't big fans either.)

After the Civil War in the South, Blacks were empowered and many southern whites were denied the right to vote. This short-lived spasm lasted until the carpetbaggers pulled out in the 1870s, when not too surprisingly, things went back to "normal." (The vote was doing just ducky in New York though, where in 1868 and '72, about 10% more people voted than were eligible. The Empire state has always been *so* progressive.)

The next and last great populist wave came in the FDR years when women and immigrants, spurred on by radio, gave us our closest approximation to democracy—apologies to most Blacks, Latinos and Native Americans, of course.

Since then it's been one step forward and two steps back as money has enhanced its partnership with power, to the detriment of the vote, as the primary currency of elected office.

A License to Steal

Today, after two centuries of reform upon reform, the system is more corrupt than ever. **Legalized profiteering** is a more apt description of our political system than representative democracy. We have a capitalistic system of commerce, all well and good; but we also have a capital driven government which is not so good. There are no more important, or sadly bankrupt, words in our Constitution than the charge to our government in the Preamble to "promote the general welfare."

Ours is a government driven by the power and money of special interests. Attention paid to promotion of the general welfare is of the cover-your-ass, throw-em-a-bone, time-to-cap-the-fangs-and-give-em-a-smile variety.

People waste their lives in myriad conservative/liberal death struggles when all they are fighting for are jive-assed bragging rights and the few coins that fall off the back of the heisted armored truck with our tax dollars inside. Politicians live for this charade. The more people can be set against one another, the easier it is for them to divvy the pie unmolested.

The Power of the Purse

That's not to say that there aren't real consequences to who wins elections, and semi-real advocates on certain issues. It is very important to Democrats and Republicans who wins elections, and who holds the balance of power in our various levels of government.

This for you neophytes is known as "the power of the purse."

For example, when Democrats win in Atlanta, it usually means millions of dollars in added commissions for the "non-profit" corporations that administer much of Atlanta's low cost housing, medical care, and rehab programs. These corporations are, almost invariably, profitably tied to an urban Democratic machine.

When Republicans win in Pennsylvania, some of those same money spigots slam shut in Philly and Pittsburgh. This doesn't create some great windfall for the people in the Keystone state. Instead it's the same budget crunch, while tax reform benefits the wealthy, and privatization contracts that enrich a few cost many their livelihoods.

At the federal level the power of the purse has taken truly mythic proportions. Electoral victory spells literally billions of dollars diverted to special interests that used to line up primarily on one side of the aisle, or the other. Today, special interests carefully cover their bets by funding both parties. Democrats and Republicans don't mind. It's still the same game for them; there's just more money. Winning, whether the Presidency or majorities in Congress, means that they get to collect most of the special interest commissions, and send more folks through the revolving door of private sector access and public sector influence. The only losers are the American people, whose vote is constantly diminished by the rising tide of money.

The Money Pit

Washington D.C., the phantasmagorical land of smoke and distorted mirrors, makes Alice's Wonderland look like some benign utopia. Who can tell who's who or what's what? Money pours into Washington from everywhere, all the time. In many ways, Israelis and Kuwaitis, per capita, are better represented in Washington than Americans because of the enormous amount of cash they funnel into it.

Ronald Reagan was paid two million dollars for making a few speeches in Japan immediately after leaving the presidency. This was more money than he received from the American people for being their president for eight years—eight years in which he talked tough to the Japanese about our trade deficit, but little was ever done. When he took the money, no one in Washington even blinked. It was just business as usual.

Some major corporations have more influence in Washington than our major cities. Executives of the Bechtel Corporation, the international construction monolith, have enjoyed revolving door employment on the cabinet of every Republican president since Eisenhower.

The military and their contractors may have as much influence as everyone else put together when it comes time to cut up the American pie. Today, in a world where a starving North Korea and a defeated Iraq are held as our greatest threats, we maintain a nuclear arsenal capable of destroying the whole planet several times over.

One last example. Head Start has been called "the motherhood and apple pie of Government programs." Everybody is crazy about it—the President and parents, Congress and local politicians of every persuasion, yet after years of proven success, it remains less than 50% funded. Why? Because, lacking the advocacy of big dollars pumped into our *electoral* system, poor children cannot compete.

As Jerry Brown, California's infamous Governor Moonbeam, so clearly stated:

> The insatiable appetite for campaign dollars has turned the government into a stop and shop for every greedy and narrow interest.
>
> The quid pro quo could not be any more straightforward. The legality of the barter cannot mask its inherent corruptness. Nor can any degree of dissembling obscure the truth that this bargain has been executed—almost without exception—to the detriment of the national interest and at the expense of the American people.

This my friends is the Mother of all Velox overlays when it comes to understanding our politics. So, unless and until a minor miracle happens and the value of the vote is finally elevated above the power of the dollar in our electoral process, if you can't vote with a BIG checkbook it doesn't mean a whole helluva lot.

What Can Be Done

An early reader of this book commented that I was just like all of the other old folks. "You tell us what's wrong, but don't tell us how to fix it."

It is a fair point, though not my intention. What I have attempted to do is to write about how the world is, not what is wrong with it. (The fact that there seems to be a lot of overlap is just an inconvenient coincidence.) Two primary thoughts drove this decision. First, that accurate information, or at least as accurate as one muddled brain could offer, was pretty valuable in our "strings attached" world. Second, because I was "should on" way too much when younger, I wasn't going to continue the pathology.

One of the reader's primary complaints was the lack of an offered solution in "Politics." As I thought about the suggestion, weighing the intimation that I was "just like all of the other old folks," against the slippery slope of a little well-intentioned should-ing, I saw a perfectly bad lose/lose situation. I will try to meet him halfway, though, by saying what I believe needs to be done (Note the "I believe" statement, it is *an opinion*), without hazarding a guess on how to do it. I have no clue if it can be done, how it will be done, or how long it will take—ten years or a thousand years. What has led me to this decision is the idea that the legitimate progression of human governance leads to an ever greater faith in each individual to take full responsibility for his or her thoughts and actions—toward full and equal citizenship in a democracy.

As they used to say in the old gangster movies, "Here goes nuttin."

One of the Mount Rushmore boys once said, "When democracy fails, use more democracy." Judging from the rest of his work, this was probably just some 4th of July drivel, but he did say the right thing then. Like most of the rest of his buds since then, however, he kept getting the oral-anal thing confused when it came to 'WE the people.'

The "I Got Mine" Crowd

The opponents of democracy are an (often unwitting) league of haves and elites (and yes, there is a generous crossover between the two). We know why the haves don't want too much democracy. They worry that with the poorer majority in charge, their taxes will rise.

Elites are a little different story. They require a more careful examination. I'm using the term elite to define our professional class: doctors, lawyers, architects, business executives, clergy, engineers, and PhDs of all sorts. I'm not disparaging the work they do. It is obviously important. In their particular specialties, it is their job to know what is best. In their particular fields they are the experts. These experts, however, too often think that because they are elite in one way, they are elite in other ways. When they think this, they are usually wrong. Does a medical doctor know more than a house painter about our political system? Will an architect make more informed decisions about promoting the general welfare of the country than a waitress? My experience is that professional expertise hard earned in one discipline has little value outside that particular specialty. Very often, a waitress who reads the paper and stays interested in goings-on will make the more informed decision.

It is with regard to elected governance that the problem magnifies. Elites too often think that they know what is best for the rest of us. They believe that their superior education, training, and insight as to the ways that things are really done gives them some reasoned advantage over the rest of us, gives them a reason to act as our wise surrogates. This might be fine if it was done after the election, at the request of the elected. Elites in America too often skip the fair election part. They, like old Al Hamilton, often don't trust the commoner to do the right thing. This is why they aren't on the bandwagon to promote the equal value of each and every vote. The feeling is that us common folk are too easily led, too capricious, and not discerning enough for true responsibility.

I disagree.

Human Nature

Human potential is incredibly broad in both directions. If you expect the worst from us, don't respect or trust us, treat us poorly, and give us little incentive to improve, we can exceed your worst expectations. However, if you treat us with simple dignity, trust us to act responsibly in our own best interest, and give us the opportunity, we will rarely disappoint.

Truth is, the whole argument should be moot. We are supposed to be a democracy. It's our thing, what we're famous for. That, and capitalism. Most everybody here believes in democracy and capitalism.

So how come we only have capitalism? Fortunately, I bored you with those details earlier. Though we still talk about more democracy, little is ever actually done to promote its reality.

"Kiss My Campaign-Finance-Reformed Ass"

Today_____(fill in the date) our politicians are talking about campaign finance reform. "Campaign finance reform" is an illusion. Our present system is an example of extensive reform.

Campaign finance reform is fatally flawed because of its lower status legally when weighed against our free speech rights. The Constitution gives all Americans the right to almost total freedom of speech. The big exceptions involve immediate public safety, like yelling "Fire!" in a crowded theater, or inciting a gathering of people into a murderous mob. Beyond that, and other types of physically abusive language, no one can stop you from saying whatever you want to say.

Usually this is a good thing. When combined with great wealth in our electoral process, however, it quickly robs most people of the equal value of their vote, and equal entry to elected office.

Our vote is diminished because campaign finance laws cannot stop a wealthy person from circumventing legal donation limits to a candidate or party. The Free Speech Amendment in the Constitution overrides this, guaranteeing an individual's right to spend as much money as he or she wants to personally advocate for a candidate, or for an issue closely associated with a candidate.

If you use your vote, and someone else uses his or her vote, and a lot of money, they have more say in the election. Call it what you like. It ain't democracy.

Similarly, if you want to run for office, the person with just a good rap is disadvantaged if running against someone else with a good line of BS *and* lots of cash to advertise it.

Campaign finance reform is analogous to building a dam halfway across a river—it doesn't work. It only works to keep most of us thinking that something is being done. Something is being done. It is being done *to* us, however, rather than *for* us.

To Mend You Must Amend

Unfortunately, the only way for the United States to become a true democracy is to amend our Constitution, to elevate the importance of each individual vote. Recent Supreme Court decisions, based on the Free Speech Amendment in the Bill of Rights, preclude any action that would reduce an individual's right to spend his or her own money in support of a candidate for elective office. What is needed is a stronger amendment aimed strictly at our electoral process that would elevate the value of the individual vote above the power of money (in the months prior to an election). The right to have each person's franchise count equally must be placed above an individual's "free speech" right to spend as much money as he or she wants in support of a candidate.

Imagining

Geez, imagine that. Imagine living in a country where your vote counted just as much as the rich folks'. Where a rich idiot like Steve Forbes couldn't spend $50 million trying to sucker us into a tax break for the rich, or where another rich idiot couldn't spend another 50 mil trying to sell us on his Napoleonic complex. Imagine a country where our political leaders don't have to be hosed down every hour to remove the bullshit that oozes from their pores. Imagine that.

Imagining you can do something is the first step toward accomplishing it.

The next individual step is to think and talk about a purer democracy. What are the ramifications? Is greater democracy a step too far, or is it a natural evolutionary step in human governance? Is it really foolish to trust the common people with equal say in a complex world, or is true democracy just what we need to keep the greedy folks, xenophobics, bullshit artists, and bullies more in line? Will it solve more problems than it creates? Is it an idea whose time has come? Is it overdue, or is it still premature? Can it be done? How might that happen? What would be different? What would be the same?

Don't take my word for it, or anybody else's. Check it out for yourself. If moving toward greater democracy is a good thing, the right thing, it will begin to take on a life of its own. Shakespeare coined a phrase for what may be the most effective weapon in human conflict: He called it hoisting folks on their own petard. The petard of hypocrites is their own lies and half truths. You can use their own words and ideas to show the error of their ways, to point out their hypocrisy.

Hoisting hypocrites on their own petard works great.

If we call ourselves a democracy, how come most people only have a vote in an election, while others can vote and donate lots of money? If most folks would like Head Start to be fully funded, why don't we build a few less bombers and use the extra money to fully fund Head Start? This is a democracy, isn't it? Or do the people that make a lot of money building bombers really count more than poor kids?

There's a tough one.

Rock, Paper & Scissors

This is a game I learned as a child. It is played with one other person by each simultaneously shooting out a hand as either a fist (symbolizing a rock), a flat hand (= paper), or with your index and middle finger separated (indicating a pair of scissors). In the game rock breaks scissors, scissors cuts paper, and paper covers rock.

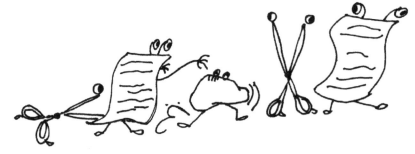

Much later I realized that Rock, Paper & Scissors was a metaphor for humans in contrast. Someone was always better than someone else at something. In other things, someone else would be better. Occasionally rock-paper-scissors happens when people are competing at the same thing: A has B's number, B has C's, but C handles A. I love it when that happens.

The lasting wisdom of rock-paper-scissors lies in the futility of egoistic comparison. There is usually someone better, prettier, smarter, stronger, tougher, and someone further down these comparative totem poles. So what. It's all just a game of rock-paper-scissors. Don't waste your time.

Drugs

If Shakespeare were alive and coming of age today, he would have probably uttered more than a few "Forsooths" over the dilemma of drugs in today's society. It is a very complicated subject:

> To take drugs, or not to take drugs,
> That is the question.

That, and which ones to take or not to take, which combinations to take or not to take them in, and when to take or not take them; which of course is just the beginning. You can also wind up in pressure-inducing scenes, then on top of complication there's compression. "What are ya gonna do," "Cmon, hurry up!" " Make up your mind." Drugs often attract pressure: peer, parental, police. Makes you wonder if some folks don't start taking drugs just to relieve some of the drug-induced pressure. How's a person supposed to make good decisions about drugs when there's **so much Goddamn PRESSURE?!!**

It is not easy. Remembering that you are the star of this show, though, is a good place to start. Don't allow anyone to pressure you into taking, or doing, anything you don't want to. You decide what to put, or not to put, in your body. This is the best drug law that there is.

This, of course, is all predicated on some sort of passing into adulthood. While individuals should decide for themselves what to do with their own bodies and lives, you have to get through the childhood—growing-up—dependency thing before the I—me—mine rights fully kick in. For most, between 18 and 21 is that time range, though some few of us are earlier or later bloomers to personal responsibility. Here is a fairly reliable marker for this: When you have assumed total responsibility for yourself and your actions in this world, you are ready to decide for yourself what is best for you.

Deciding what is best for you can be pretty complicated too, unless you take an all or nothing approach, and even the nothing approach has several variations. There's the very chaste "Nothing will pass these pristine lips, and anyone who takes drugs ought to be in jail" route. Then there are the "straight edge," hard-core people who like to live out on the edge and don't want anything distorting by even a little bit where that precarious edge might be. And there are other folks that for whatever good and appropriate reasons prefer to leave off temporal alteration at the exigencies of soda pop, singing, meditation, or just breathing sweet air. With the possible exception of the pass-judgement types, **All Perfectly Cool**. On the other end there's the extremely liberal "Gimme anything you've got" Air Gonzo approach.

OK, now that we've narrowed the parameters, let's talk.

People who do take drugs usually take them because these drugs make them feel good. Problem is, it's hard to know when to stop. If a little of a drug makes you feel a little better, so the logic goes, a lot should make you feel fantastic; but like cake and ice cream when we were kids, eventually too much can make us sick.

It's hard to decide what to talk about and what not to. Some folks make some pretty bizarre decisions in life, and drugs seem to be an especially vulnerable area. I'm generally assuming a modicum of sanity in the reader, so those who are into flaming airplane glue, turpentine and Drano cocktails will have to look for guidance elsewhere. I am not talking about antibiotics, aspirin, Tylenol, or trying to get off on three tiny little time pills either. By the time most of you are ready to read this you have avoided or moved beyond the illusory temptations of cough syrup, glue, whipped cream and other household inhalants. Medicine to regulate organ function and blood pressure, whether high or low, will mostly just make you feel weird, a state that many of us here in Babylon have little trouble attaining drug free. Anyway, rummaging around Granny's medicine cabinet (while she's still alive), is not only extremely rude; it's not very promising.

Drugs and The Law

Drug laws are culturally driven. Different cultures have differing laws. Generally the more mono-dogmatic and -chromatic a culture, the stricter the drug prohibitions; the more tolerant and accepting of difference a culture is, the more liberal the laws. We're somewhere in the middle here in the U S of A. We have all manner of differences here. We're just not all that tolerant of them.

Drugs are our last great scapegoat. We can't blame our problems on the Commies anymore, and less easily now on women, minorities, or homosexuals. And God knows we're not going to start blaming the real culprits. Democracy, unlike Catholicism, has no confessional.

Much of our national drug-taking philosophy stems from the age-appropriateness of drugs. Drugs are very age appropriate. Most of our lawmakers are 40 & up. The drug of choice for that age group is alcohol. Hence alcohol is legal and plentiful.

Alcohol and marijuana are on either side of the legal line in the sand that our society has drawn. The formula for drawing it is a little complicated but not that hard to follow. They are both known as gateway drugs, meaning that they can lead to more dangerous drugs. The problem with this theory is that alcohol addiction is hugely damaging by itself. Between ten and twenty percent (depending on your statistical source) of those who begin drinking become alcoholics. "Reefer Madness" is primarily projected uptight hysteria. People who smoke too much pot have more in common with people who eat too many potato chips and watch too much TV. They become, shall we say, vegetative. This would seem to weigh on the side of making pot legal and alcohol illegal, but of course there is more.

Alcohol is the great eraser. That's why the old folks are so fond of it. It is both a numbant and a dumbant. The older you get, generally, the more set in your ways you become. The more set in your ways you become the more disoriented you get, because you lose the flexibility of changing as new and better information comes to you. Eventually, *you* become the problem. If alcohol is your drug of choice, it not only won't remind you of this, it will conveniently help you to forget it. Pot, on the other hand, alters perspective without the anesthesia. It is psycho active. In moderation it generally nudges you toward new, and sometimes expanded thinking. The marijuana high is very upsetting to old folks, it rocks their artificial world, brings in too much reality at once, stirs up too much stuff. If it does this for them, it will do it for their kids, and "We don't need no crazy pot smokin hippies rockin our boat." So alcohol is perfectly legal and the ganja got to be smoked on de sly, mon.

The Bad Shit

I'm not going to spend a lot of time on this. If you can get the drift of what I'm saying in this book, crack cocaine, crystal Methedrine, and in generally descending order, speed, heroin, the designer hallucinogens, barbiturates, coke and any other crap that can create your very own Hellboundtrain, is not going to be too enticing to you. If it is, put this book to much better use, and beat the hell out of yourself with it.

What's worse: crack, heroin or speed?

What's worse: killing yourself and a friend, killing yourself and a family member, or maiming yourself and killing three strangers?

What I'm saying here is that: **They Are <u>All</u> FUCKED UP!!!**

"Different Strokes for Different Folks"

One of the problems in talking about drugs is that people have such differing reactions to them. One person's whiskey is another's tea. You generally have to figure this out for yourself, although that doesn't mean that you have to personally make extensive field tests of every Controlled Dangerous Substance and their possible combinations to see what floats and what sinks your boat. Being cautious is a good idea. A lot of boats, once they sink, that's it. Even if someone refloats your sunk boat, you can have some pretty permanent water damage. I've known lots of folks with permanent "water damage." I've also known some people that are a different kind of mess because they've been too paranoid to see if their boat floated.

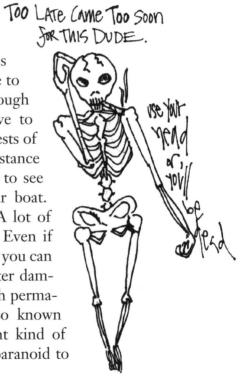

Too Late Came Too Soon for This Dude.

use your head or, you'll be dead

It used to be that a high tolerance for alcohol was an important attribute in society. Can you *hold* your liquor? The macho drinking contest has been a big part of the cultural mosaic here and world-wide for a couple of thousand years now. It belongs on the slag heap with a lot of the other shit we used to think was cool. If you can't drink much without getting loaded, and don't, there are lots of benefits. You are a cheap drunk, you don't beat your body up too much, you're less likely to get DWI'd, and you can still have an intelligent conversation with that person at the party that you *really* like. On the other hand, if you somehow get trapped on a tramp steamer with a bunch of cut-throat rat bastards, being able to do 42 shots of tequila may save you from having to walk the plank.

Smoking the Gange

This is a topic that I have a feeling coming-of-agers are somewhat familiar with. If not, NORML (National Association for the Reform of Marijuana Laws) at 1001 Connecticut Avenue, NW, Suite 1010, Washington, DC 20036, has wonderfully complete information on cannabis and its human applications.

Smoking marijuana is called lots of things, primarily "Getting

High." Other popular terms are "Getting Stoned," "Getting Wasted," and "Getting Wrecked." These terms are instructive. The vast majority of marijuana-induced experiences fall within these parameters.

Lots of pot smokers smoke too much. It's back to that too much of a good thing stuff. Reefer *can* be a crutch. The folks who don't think so are the folks who are definitely smoking too much. People who smoke pot recreationally, in the right places at the right times, need no advice. Enjoy. Some folks who don't smoke pot probably ought to, but they have to come to that, or not, on their own. It's always about your own individual balance. These are things you've just got to figure out for yourself.

Drug Etiquette

Most drug etiquette is simpler to learn than the more formal kinds of etiquette. There is generally more room for error. Usually if you slip up, either no one notices, or they think it's funny as hell. There are a few rules though, that *should* (I hate using that word, but this is the right time and place) be followed, stoned or sober.

- Never try to persuade someone to take a drug if they have never taken it before.

- Don't do what you don't think you can handle. By the time you realize that you can't, it is way too late.

- Never put another person at risk with your drug-related stupidity.

- Don't get caught with more than you're willing to pay for. The Man don't play that.

Anyone who is smart enough to deal drugs and make money is smart enough to make more money doing something legal. Believe it or not, that's where the money is. Anyone who's not smart enough to deal, and does, will take a fall. There is something to be said for honest dealing, but even honest dealing is a crap shoot. Don't play craps with your life.

Sex, DRUGS & Rock N Roll

Nothing is more fun than dancin, drinkin, jokin and tokin, reel-in with de feelin, and lovin all night long. Don't get hurt, don't get diseased, and don't get caught. Partying when you're a young adult can be as good as things get. Some folks believe that you can have just as good of a time without anyone getting high. Maybe you can, I'm not sure. I guess I'm not a good person to talk about that. I do know that it's fun to be at a good party where everyone else is getting high or stoned and you are straight. Not so much because you get to watch everyone make a fool of themselves, although that can be a lot of fun too. But it's great if you can get out of your inhibitions, get into the flow and get to it *au naturel.*

Drugs, like most things, are pretty self-balancing in life. Get too high on alcohol, you will feel sick the next day. This is a good general example, although each drug, or each combination of drugs, has its own individual complications. Getting high is usually followed by getting low. Often sleep can ameliorate this. Something that gets you real high is either very dangerous, will later bring you way down, or both.

Smoking a joint in the privacy of your home is **not** a crime. Almost anything done by *consenting adults* in privacy is **not** a crime. Random drug testing without probable cause is a crime. Says all of this right in the Constitution.

That's about all I feel comfortable saying. Anyone who attempts to talk rationally about drugs in our society without spewing out the preposterously convoluted party line encourages the wrath of a paranoid, lock-step status quo. I wouldn't want to be accused of "Incite to light," when my only real offense is, "Incite to think for yourself"—a high enough crime as it is in this here society.

I Am An American Patriot

I am an American patriot.

I am a free person. I think for myself.

I don't like to pledge allegiance or wave the flag. I distrust anyone who would wrap themselves in the flag.

I believe in the ideals of America, foremost, that ALL men and women are created equally, and with certain inalienable rights. Among those rights are the freedoms enumerated in our Bill of Rights, equal justice, privacy in the home and person, and a democratic process that holds sacred one vote for each person. I don't believe that these ideals end at my doorstep, or are just for a privileged few, or that they even stop at the borders of this country. As this is one nation under God, I am called upon to support these ideals for all of God's children, for all of humanity.

I strive to defend these rights for everyone, regardless of race, religion, ethnicity, gender, age, sexual orientation, or physical or mental ability, and especially for those who are least able to defend themselves.

I am egalitarian; I would never presume to be better than anyone else, and don't think that anyone else is better than me.

I was once called by my country to serve in a foreign war, and I did. The cause I was called to serve in was unjust. We were sent to a country to impose our will on the people who lived there. It turned out that they were the patriots defending their country. These people suffered horribly, but finally prevailed as our great country lost the heart for this unjust war. It was a victory for them and a victory for the American ideal: Nobody has the right to come into your country and impose their will on you.

No one has the right to wrap himself in a flag of patriotism to oppress you.

If my country calls me again, I will not respond so quickly. I might find that my patriotic duty calls on me to resist with every fiber of my being. If it is a just cause, I will proudly serve again.

I also believe the United States is supposed to be a noble meritocracy. This is something we have gotten too far away from.

As a child growing up in America, my role was quite clear to me. All children started out even here, and were given an equal chance to succeed. My success in life would be determined by my own conduct, like all of the other children. In school, in church, or in other activities it didn't matter who your parents were, or how much money they had. What mattered was what you did, and how you did it.

Were I to be successful, the privilege earned would bring with it corresponding obligations of service to those less able, and to the country as a whole. By action and through example, the more able, ascended through achievement, assured freedom and justice for all.

It is to these American ideals that I freely give my allegiance.

Feminine Facial Hair
& Other Imperfections

As a young man, I was full of petty prejudices that it has taken much of my adult life to shed. One of the absolute worst of these afflictions was my aversion to feminine facial hair.

A young woman could be attractive to me in every way, but if she had the remotest shadow visible above her lip, she might as well have been a leper. This sad state of affairs followed me around for many years. When added to all my other self-defeating baggage, it's amazing I was able to move around at all.

Finally at some new lonely low, I reached out to a fuzzy-faced young woman. It was partly, I am sure, to rid myself of another demon.

Well 'lo and behold'—as they say—she became a great love of my life, my most appreciative and intimate lover. Once I got past my perfect-faced prejudice, I was able to see her whole fine package. We had many wonderful times together. Sadly, the relationship had other more substantive imperfections and, like so many passionate romances, we gradually exploded apart.

I don't think there is much definitive to say about feminine facial hair or other perceived human imperfections. Everyone is imperfect. Generally the less imperfect a person is, the more removed they are from the rest of us in the muddling masses of humanity. (I'm saying that this is not necessarily good, you understand.)

Some folks are so bothered with their imperfections that they have them painfully and expensively modified. Why not? Improving your physical appearance is as worthwhile an effort as improving most other things we are constantly trying to improve. God knows we all crave and are improved by love, and whatever else might be true, physical attraction is a big part of love. Smart guy Al Einstein didn't marry a show girl for her knowledge of nuclear physics, but for her delivery of nuclear nookey.

On the other hand, physical attraction has infinite variety. Most folks have a pretty good innate sense of who they are, and from that sense, and lots of other stuff, flows a generally rational—usually attainable—idea of the type of mate that attracts them. *Attraction* is the mate magnet. Your physical imperfections, once accepted and assimilated, often make you ***more attractive***. If you work hard to improve what you can about yourself, and then have the courage to accept the rest of you as being the best that can be made of an imperfect situation, you can become quite an attractive package. Just add love and watch the whole thing bloom.

The lesson for me is to work on my own prejudices. I was robbing myself, and maybe some other nice people, of a little joy. Take it from me, joy is better than prejudice any old day.

Some Closing Thoughts

When I was a coming-of-ager in the late 60s and early 70s, many of us felt that we would be the generation to lead society out of ignorance and its accompanying jealousies and paranoias. We would correct the injustices of racism, male dominance, the fallacy of European culture as right or normative, and move toward a loving sexuality that valued everyone. We had answers, we knew we were right about everything, we were brimming with energy. Unfortunately we were ultimately full of our own, and still full of everyone else's, shit. As we've grown older my generation's shit level has risen, not fallen, as has every generation's to come through before and after us.

There are lots of reasons why my generation of hip hippies failed. We threw that old baby out with the bath water. Old was bad. New was good. Not. We thought we had all of the answers. Obviously we did not. We didn't respect the complexity of things. We didn't understand that most of life is evolutionary rather than revolutionary. We were mostly privileged kids who grew up in a distorted bubble of reality. Not having spent much time out of that bubble, we mistook it for the whole reality. Sadly, many of us still do.

There are many overwhelming reasons why each bright, shiny, energetic generation gets ground down into a "go-along, get-along" complicity with a deadening status quo. Human nature has a lot of intrinsic baggage. The herd instinct is huge. It is powerful human nature to find security not in integrity, but in numbers. The majority sides with the winners, not with those who are necessarily right. Our loyalties co-opt us. If we buy into anything besides a steady quest for justice and a common understanding, we begin to forfeit someone's right to a just world.

Each generation, as it comes along, must accept and make the best of the hand it is dealt. Reality's mosaic is always in flux. Individuals in any generation can find the bright light of truth and follow it, but every now and then the stars line up for a lucky generation of kids, and there is a renewal of truth-seeking that allows for many more to participate in finding that enlightenment. This present generation of Gen Xers, and the now following Generation Why, are similarly blessed with good birth timing.

The fortune of opportunity is double-edged with responsibility. Many in my generation eventually fell back into a womb of denial and hypocrisy. But we are uneasy in that double standard. We have glimpsed the truth. We know there is better. Maybe, in that sense, we did not fail. Believe me, we are not as hard of a nut to crack as our parents were, or as much of an obstacle to your dreams. So pursue your dreams. Pursue them with a withering honesty and respect for yourself and the world around you.

Remember that no one is better or worse than anyone else. I strive to respect even assholes who seemingly don't deserve it because, if I am honest with myself I realize, if dealt their same lousy hand, I would be that same lousy asshole.

Don't hold being old against the old, or buy into the new just because it is new. Find the best combination and make something better.

Don't worry about survival. "Existence is a good person's purse, and a bad person's keep." Have the courage to do what you think is best. You won't starve to death, and "Way will open."

Be open to other people's truths. The most valuable thing to find out is what you are most wrong about. But you are the last arbiter of that truth; trust your own truth as best for you.

Take your time.

I hope that you are able to find a mate. There is no better way to pass through this life than with a loving, respecting, and mutually supportive partner. You get to share a whole other life, to have someone who wants to share in your hopes and dreams, to lovingly glory in your accomplishments and sustain you through your failures. Of course being in a relationship where you or your partner are cheating is just so much crap. True love is founded upon true living. The degree to which you cheat life will be eventually mirrored in the dysfunction of your romance, and in any family that ensues. True living eventually equates with true romance. Most people don't realize until too late—and too late usually comes too soon—that bad clone will catch up with you. The older you get the more easily caught you become, so read what Fay Weldon has to say on the next page. She knows.

I thank you very much for reading my book and I wish you well.

"You end up as you deserve. In old age, you must put up with the face, the friends, the health and the children you have earned."

Fay Weldon

Index

*To order additional copies of
"Coming of Age in Babylon"
see order form
on the following page.*

Coming of Age in Babylon
Order Form

Fax: 609-279-0014

Phone: 800-883-7407 (Please have credit card # ready)

E-mail nwspring@bellatlantic.net

Postal Orders: New Spring Publications
                   P O Box 7632
                   Princeton, NJ 08540

Please send _____ copy/copies @ $12.00 each to:

_____

_____

_____

_____

_____

Sales Tax: Please add 6% sales tax for books shipped to New Jersey.

Shipping: Add $2.00 for first book and $1.00 for each additional book.

Payment: ❏ Check   Credit Card: ❏ VISA   ❏ MasterCard

   Card Number: _____

   Name on card: _____

   Expiration Date: _____